The Doctor's Internet Handbook

By Robert Kiley MSc ALA

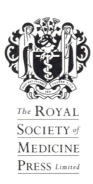

The ROYAL
SOCIETY *of*
MEDICINE
PRESS *Limited*

Contents

PREFACE   v

CHAPTER ONE   How to get medical information from the Internet   1

CHAPTER TWO   Current awareness services on the Internet   7

CHAPTER THREE   Medical databases on the Internet: part 1   13

CHAPTER FOUR   Medical databases on the Internet: part 2   19

CHAPTER FIVE   Internet discussion lists   25

CHAPTER SIX   Evidence-based medicine on the Internet   31

CHAPTER SEVEN   Medical journals on the World Wide Web   35

CHAPTER EIGHT   Consumer health information on the Internet   41

CHAPTER NINE   Health statistics on the World Wide Web   47

CHAPTER TEN   Medical education on the World Wide Web   51

CHAPTER ELEVEN   Quality of medical information on the Internet   57

CHAPTER TWELVE   The Internet and healthcare — the future   63

CHAPTER THIRTEEN   Endpiece   67

INDEX   73

Preface

A recent survey into usage of the Internet amongst GPs found that the principal reason for getting connected was the desire to obtain up-to-date clinical information, particularly from online medical journals and other information sources such as MEDLINE[1]. Once connected to the Internet however, most GPs reported that the biggest problem they faced was trying to find relevant information in a timely and efficient manner. Indeed, with the number of pages on the World Wide Web now thought to total more than 275 million—with an additional 20 million pages being created every month—this problem is one which is readily understood[2].

This book attempts to mitigate this problem by providing the busy doctor with a wealth of information on useful and relevant Web sites. Arranged thematically, the book covers topics such as current awareness services, medical databases and consumer health information. Coverage is also given to the crucial subjects of quality and evidence-based medicine, whilst the introductory chapter provides information on how to search effectively for medical information on the Internet.

Originally published in the *Journal of the Royal Society of Medicine*, these articles have been revised and updated for this new publication. This book also has a supporting Web site which contains hypertext links to all the sites discussed herein. Not only does this mean that *all* sites can be reached from a single source but, more importantly, if a URL (the Web address) changes this can be reflected on this page, thus ensuring that all sites remain reachable. To access the home page of the *Doctor's Guide to the Internet Handbook* point your Web browser at: http://www.roysocmed.ac.uk/handbook.htm

ROBERT KILEY

Information Service Manager, Wellcome Trust, London, UK

REFERENCES

1   <URL: http://www.nop.co.uk/internet/surveys/pr19.htm> [Accessed 22 August 1998]

2   <URL: http://www.research.digital.com/SRC/whatsnew/sem.html> [Accessed 22 August 1998]

How to get medical information from the Internet

SEARCHING THE INTERNET

Despite the complexity of the Internet, most novices are pleasantly surprised how easy it is to search for information. Both the *Netscape Navigator* and the *Microsoft Internet Explorer* — the two most popular Web browsers — have a 'Net Search' button. Clicking this button takes you to a Web page where you can either run a search on a chosen Internet database — *Netscape* currently points to AltaVista — or select another search engine from a reasonably exhaustive list. Either way, searching for a subject simply requires the user to input a word or phrase in the search-box, and press the 'Enter' key.

When you are looking for health/medical information, however, the shortcomings associated with this method of searching soon become all too evident.

- You find too much. A search for information on 'asthma' on the AltaVista search engine identifies some 94 800 potentially relevant Internet sites.

- You find irrelevant material. A search of AltaVista for 'migraine' suggests that the most relevant Web site is 'Migraine Boy' — a cartoon character (see Figure 1.1).

- You find inaccurate and misleading information. A search for 'Melatonin' identifies numerous Web sites where the qualities of this drug are described. The Quality Health Inc Web site — a mail order pharmaceutical business in the UK — describes this drug in the following manner:

Well known as a treatment for jet lag and insomnia, numerous studies are being conducted to investigate whether Melatonin has anti-ageing and anti-cancer properties[1].

Warnings about this drug are restricted to the simple caution that you should not drive or operate machinery after taking. Nowhere are the possible adverse effects — fragmented sleep patterns, headaches, mild depression — even hinted at[2–5].

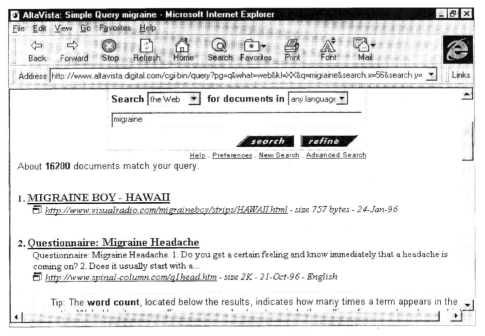

Figure 1.1 **A search for migraine at AltaVista**

FINDING GOOD QUALITY HEALTH INFORMATION ON THE INTERNET

To help you find high quality medical information on the Internet several specialty search services have been developed. The most relevant of these are discussed below.

Health on the Net
(http://www.hon.ch)

The Health on the Net Foundation is a non-profit organization dedicated to 'realising the benefits of the Internet and related technologies in the fields of medicine and healthcare'.

To meet this objective the Foundation has developed a Code of Conduct for medical and health Web sites. Central to this code is the principle that medical information must 'only be given by medically trained and qualified professionals'. When this condition cannot be met there must be 'a clear statement...that a piece of advice offered is from a non-medically qualified individual'. Internet sites which comply with this code are granted the right to display the Health on the Net logo on their pages. In time it is hoped that this logo will represent a stamp of quality, in much the same way as the BS5750 kite mark does.

Surprisingly, though, the searchable database of Internet resources is *not* limited to those sites which comply with the Code. Indeed, a search of the database identifies three distinct types of data:

1   Resources that comply with the Code

2   Resources that do *not* comply with the Code but have been reviewed by the Health on the Net team

3   Resources that do *not* comply with the Code and have *not* been reviewed. (Resources in this section are compiled from 'recommendations' from those Web sites which comply with the HON Code.)

Moreover, it would be a mistake to assume that only those sites which complied with the Code were worth using. When searching the database for UK resources—a useful feature when so much of the Net has a US bias—I found that, though the British Diabetic Association and the Cancer Research Centre Web sites are 'Code compliant', the *BMJ*, the Department of Health and the Medicines Control Agency Web sites are not.

Overall, I believe that development of a quality Code of Conduct is a valuable contribution to the evolution of medical information on the Internet. However, until the Code becomes more widely recognized—and perhaps the *de facto* standard—the Health on the Net site will remain a resource amongst many others that health professionals will have to use. The much-sought-after 'one-stop shop' has yet to arrive.

Medical Matrix
(http://www.medmatrix.org/index.asp)

One of the more established medical search services, the Medical Matrix Project, is 'devoted to posting, annotating, and continuously updating full content, unrestricted access, Internet clinical medicine resources'.

The Matrix currently has links to around 4000 quality assessed Internet sites, all of which reside within a browseable, hierarchical subject index. The seven top-level headings include 'Speciality and Disease Categorisation', 'Clinical Practice' and 'Education'. Within each section of the hierarchy resources are further subdivided to allow the user the opportunity to focus the enquiry. For example, oncology resources are divided into categories such as 'News', 'Clinical Trials', 'Practice Guidelines' and 'Diseases'. This last subdivision allows the user to select a more specific cancer term, such as 'breast cancer' or 'gastrointestinal tumours' (see Figure 1.2).

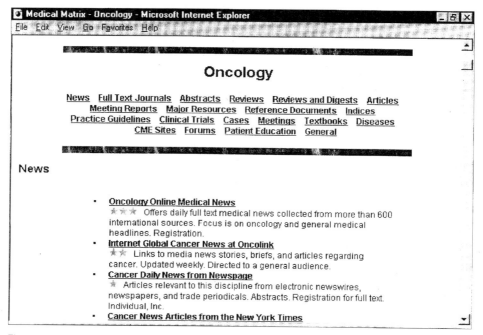

Figure 1.2   **Oncology resources at Medical Matrix**

Another useful feature of the Matrix is the ranking system it employs. Though *all* the sites within the Matrix meet the basic quality criteria — they provide specialized knowledge with suitable clinical content — sites which are deemed to be 'best of a speciality category' or 'a premier Web site for the discipline' are awarded merit stars.

Healthtel, the publishers of Matrix, insist that anyone who wishes to use the resource must complete an online registration form (the site still remains free of charge). Though form-filling may discourage some users I would urge all health professionals who are keen to find accurate high-quality health resources on the Internet to complete the registration form and exploit the resources contained with the Matrix.

OMNI — Organised Medical Networked Information
(http://www.omni.ac.uk)

Describing itself as the 'UK's gateway to high quality biomedical resources on the Internet', OMNI is another key resource for health professionals.

Like the Medical Matrix, the OMNI resources database can be both searched and browsed. Recognizing the power of browsing however, the OMNI team have developed an interface which allows the user to browse the database in three ways — by alphabetic topic, by classified topic, and by MeSH (Medical Subject Headings). This last option — derived from the NLM UMLS metathesaurus — supports broader and narrower relationships, thus allowing far more precise and focused browsing. For example, on selecting the MeSH term 'diabetes mellitus', you are given the opportunity to select a more specific term, 'diabetes mellitus — complications', a broader term, 'endocrine disorder', or a related term such as 'thyroid disease'.

To provide a focus for UK Internet resources the OMNI database, like Health on the Net, supports the option to restrict a search to UK material.

The OMNI site also has details of how resources are evaluated for inclusion in the database, plus some excellent articles relating to the quality of health information on the Internet.

CliniWeb
(http://www.ohsu.edu/cliniweb)

Developed by the Oregon Health Sciences Library, CliniWeb is another powerful tool for identifying high-quality clinical information on the Web.

Adopting an approach that is unique amongst the medical search services discussed here, CliniWeb indexes Internet resources at the level of *individual* pages. For example, whereas both OMNI and the Matrix provide a single link to the American Medical Association (AMA) Internet site, the team at CliniWeb have gone further and indexed the individual pages which exist on the AMA site. Thus, a search at CliniWeb for 'Tuberculosis' points you (amongst other things) to an article in *Archives of Pediatrics and Adolescent Medicine* on 'tuberculosis testing' and an article in *JAMA* entitled 'Risk factors for tuberculosis in HIV-infected persons'.

To assist the Internet searcher yet further, the developers of CliniWeb have written a computer program that translates natural language terms to the correct MeSH heading. Thus, 'postnatal depression' is mapped to 'depression, postpartum' and 'heart attack' to 'myocardial infarction'. This mapping facility negates the need for CliniWeb users to be fully cognizant with the intricacies of MeSH. Once a MeSH term has been identified it displays a list of Internet resources which have been indexed on that term.

The explicit commitment at CliniWeb to include *only* Internet resources that contain clinical information suitable for 'health care education or practice' ensures that searches conducted here refer health professionals to relevant and appropriate information sources.

Table 1.1 **Internet Search Services—a quick comparison**

Search service	Measles (No. of identified resources)	Diabetic retinopathy (No. of identified resources)	Database size (No. of records)	Last database update
Health on the Net	7 (+99*)	3 (+45*)	2000 (20 000*)	28 July 1997
Medical Matrix	5	1	4111	21 July 1997
OMNI	7	1	1671	15 July 1997
CliniWeb	9	6	10000	5 May 1997
AltaVista	17794	1000	31 million	Not disclosed

*These figures represent sites indexed by Health on the Net but have not yet been reviewed

Which service is best?

Table 1.1 shows the number of Internet resources that were found when two specific searches were run against the search services discussed here. All the searches were run on 28 July 1997.

With the exception of the AltaVista search engine, which has no quality filter, the numbers of resources identified by the specialized medical search services are all of the same magnitude. Of greater significance, however, was the finding that the resources identified by one search service were rarely picked up by a competitor service. The conclusion to be drawn from this finding is that if physicians want to do a *comprehensive* search for quality health resources on the Internet they must be prepared to use a range of search services.

REFERENCES

1   <URL: http://www.qhi.co.uk/product.htm> [Accessed 19 July 1997]

2   Lamberg L. Melatonin potentially useful, but safety, efficacy remain uncertain. *JAMA* 1996;**276**:1011–14

3   Ellis CM, Lemmens G, Parkes JD. Melatonin and insomnia. *J Sleep Res* 1996;**5**:61–5

4   Middleton BA, Stone BM, Arendt J. Melatonin and fragmented sleep patterns. *Lancet* 1996;**348**:551–2

5   Porter LM. Can melatonin cause severe headaches? *RN* 1996;**59**(4):75

Current awareness
services on the Internet

Keeping abreast of new developments in medicine is a time consuming task that requires considerable diligence. Indeed, if you consider that in an average month some 50 000 new citations are added to the MEDLINE database, the thought of checking out new health stories that might have appeared on the Internet is far from appealing. 'Information fatigue syndrome' is a condition most health professionals are all too aware of. The Internet, however, is the undisputed champion of current information. Even with today's modern publishing methods many weeks can elapse before research findings submitted for publication find their way into print. It takes even longer for traditional bibliographic databases to index these items. By contrast, the Internet allows instant publishing and instant retrieval.

The resources discussed below demonstrate some of the services now available on the Internet that can help health professionals keep abreast of new developments in their specialty. For clarity, I have split this discussion into three sections — personalized electronic newspapers, general health news and new research findings.

PERSONALIZED ELECTRONIC NEWSPAPERS

NewsTracker
http://nt.excite.com/

NewsPage
http://www.newspage.com/

These two services allow you to define an electronic 'newspaper' that includes *only* news stories that match search criteria you have defined.

Excite's NewsTracker searches the Web for articles several times each day, collecting thousands of articles from over 300 Web-based newspapers and magazines. Though it is not aimed exclusively at health professionals, the periodicals scanned and indexed by this service include the *New England Journal of Medicine* and the *New Scientist*, as well as newspapers such as the *Guardian*, *New York Times* and the *Washington Post*. Once you have defined your 'newspaper' — by supplying a list of relevant keywords — NewsTracker searches its database for relevant stories. Figure 2.1 shows the stories retrieved for my 'cloning newspaper'. (Keywords included 'cloning' 'dolly the sheep' and 'genes'). If, in this example, I am interested by the story on the cloned bull, clicking on the headline will bring the full story to my desktop.

One of the powerful features of this service is the way identified news stories can be used to refine and target the search strategy. This is achieved by simply checking the 'liked it' box, and mouse-clicking the 'learn what I like' button. A completely free service, NewsTracker allows you to define (and save) up to 50 separate news-search strategies.

The second news-service to consider is NewsPage. Similar in concept to NewsTracker, the NewsPage service has a more health-oriented focus. Of the 600 information sources (magazines, newsletters, newspapers, and news-wire services) scanned daily, around 85 focus on health.

Once you have registered with NewsPage you can create your newspaper by using the topic browser to select a particular subject interest. Alternatively, if these topics are too broad you can

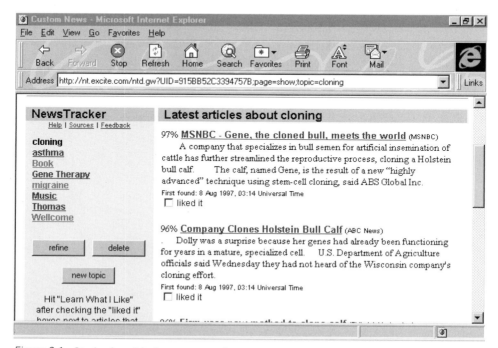

Figure 2.1 **Stories from 'cloning newspaper'**

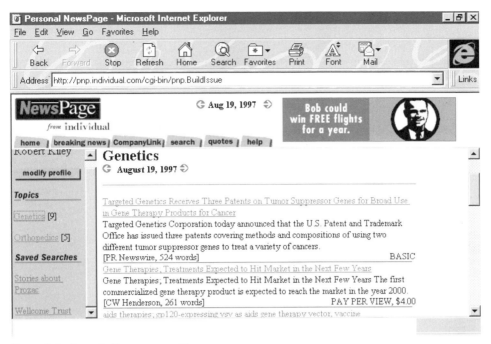

Figure 2.2 **Part of a Newspage profile**

define a more specific search — perhaps looking for information about a named drug, or a specific disease — and save this in your personal profile. Figure 2.2 shows my NewsPage profile, which consists of a mix of general topics (genetics and orthopaedics) plus some saved searches that identify stories about Prozac or the Wellcome Trust.

As with NewsTracker, no charge is made to create your NewsPage newspaper. However, in a move which I suspect will become the norm, the proprietors of NewsPage have established a fee-based system whereby certain news stories can only be viewed in full if you are prepared to pay; the headline and abstract are still free of charge. Prices of the stories vary, but a typical cost is $4 per item.

The NewsPage service also provides you with the option of receiving your daily 'newspaper' via e-mail. As this service negates the need to log-on to the NewsPage server and collect your newspaper, the fee of $3 per month seems very reasonable.

GENERAL HEALTH NEWS

Reuters Health
http://www.reutershealth.com/

Medscape
http://www.medscape.com/

Doctor's Guide
http://www.docguide.com/mednews.htm

CDPC
http://www.cdpc.com/

If you require a more *general* overview of recent health stories there are several Internet services you can call on.

The first resource worthy of mention is the Reuters Health WWW site, which provides visitors with a daily digest of health stories from around the world. Moreover, recognizing the near-universal interest in health, Reuters divide news items into stories which are of interest to health professionals and those which are more relevant to consumers. This Web site also allows you to search the text of every press release issued by Reuters Health within the past two years. For example, a search for information on 'migraine' identified around 200 news stories, the most recent of which was just 24 hours old. It is also noteworthy that all stories carried by Reuters are fully referenced. Thus, the physician reading the story headed 'Sumatriptan nasal spray is safe and well tolerated' is pointed to the source of this story, in this case an article in *Cephalalgia* (1997;**17**:541–50). Reuters Health is a subscription-based service: a one year membership costs $99.

Another way of keeping abreast of new stories is to register with Medscape, or the Doctor's Guide to the Internet, and receive, by e-mail, a weekly summary of the most important health news.

The Medscape newsletter, *Medpulse*, tends to focus on key articles which have been published within the past week, whilst the *Doctor's Guide* concentrates more on health stories that have made the news. Inevitably there is overlap between the two services, and in the week I looked to see how they compared, both had picked up some recent research on erectile dysfunction. However, whereas *Medpulse* simply reported the results of the research, the *Doctor's Guide* provided its readers with a list of other Internet sites where more information about this condition could be found. Both newsletters are supplied free of charge, and if your e-mail software is 'http enabled' (lets you link directly to a Web page) you can go straight to the Medscape or Doctor's Guide Web site and read the full text of any relevant news story.

One final news service in this section is the Communicable Disease and Prevention Control (CDPC) alerting service. The CDPC service provides summaries of infectious and communicable disease reports that are relevant for the prevention and control of these diseases. This information originates from the *Communicable Disease Reports* from the Centers for Disease Control, World Health Organization and other health agencies.

On the day I looked at this service (10 August 1997) it contained a report of a plague in Mozambique (dated the day previous) and summaries of the current issues of the *Weekly Epidemiological Report* and *Morbidity Mortality Weekly Report*, plus reports of relevant news stories from *The Lancet* and *JAMA*. No charges are made at this site.

NEW RESEARCH FINDINGS

UnCoverWeb
http://uncweb.carl.org/

WebMedLit
http://www.webmedlit.com/

Most of the resources discussed so far have focused on health stories that have been deemed newsworthy. What these services do not identify so readily are the routine, but equally important, research findings published in the world's learned medical journals.

This type of research is usually identified by a literature search on a database such as MEDLINE, with 'limiting' of results to documents added since the last update. However, in view of the time taken for MEDLINE to index articles, this database is of little value for current awareness purposes. A search of the OVID Medline database on CD-ROM, dated August 1997, reveals that the most up-to-date citation from the *BMJ* is 17 May 1997 (i.e. a 3-month gap between publication and inclusion in this database).

Two Internet services which can help plug this gap are UnCoverWeb and WebMedLit. UnCoverWeb is a database of more than seven million journal articles, drawn from nearly 17 000 English language journals; about 2500 are medical, and a full list can be found at http://uncweb.carl.org/uncover/subj/MEDICAL_.TXT. For the health professional wishing to keep up to date the important feature of UnCoverWeb is the fact that articles appear in this database at the *same time* the periodical issue reaches the news-stands. (Each day between 4000 and 5000 new citations are added to this database.) Thus, a search of this database for current information on 'osteomyelitis' finds, amongst other items, an article in the current issue of the *New England Journal of Medicine* (1997;**337**:428).

A less labour-intensive method of exploiting the resources of UnCoverWeb is to subscribe to the UnCoverWeb/Reveal automated alerting service. For an annual fee of $25 you can receive, by e-mail, the table of contents for up to 50 selected journals *and* create 25 current awareness keyword searches. Once defined, your keywords are run against the UnCoverWeb database on a weekly database. Details of any relevant articles are again mailed to you. For an additional fee a full-text copy of any article found in the UnCoverWeb database can be faxed to you. Articles cost $10 each plus a variable copyright fee.

The last service to look at in this category is WebMedLit. Describing itself as a 'medical headline service' WebMedLit provides health professionals with a one-stop shop to 23 quality medical journals including *BMJ*, *JAMA*, *Nature Medicine*, and the *Archives* series of the American Medical Association.

What differentiates WebMedLit from the countless other Web sites providing links to medical journals is its citation database. This database gives users the opportunity to search the contents of these 23 journals from one source, *and* the functionality to link directly back to the article (or abstract) at the individual journals' Web site. For example, I use WebMedLit to keep abreast of any recent articles which discuss the Internet. On running this search this week several articles were found including one titled *The Cardiology Beat*[1]. Clicking on this title took me to this specific article at *JAMA* Web site where, in this case at least, the full text was available for viewing. Equally impressive was the fact that WebMedLit identified this article, even though it had only been published within the previous 24 hours. No charges are levied by WebMedLit.

REFERENCE

1   Peters, R. The cardiology beat. *JAMA* 1997;**278**:451–2

Medical databases on the Internet: part 1

When looking for background information about a specific disease, or evidence to support a particular clinical intervention, most clinicians undertake some form of literature search[1,2]. Typically this involves a visit to the nearest medical library where you can either struggle through the bound volumes of *Index Medicus* or, more likely, use the library's CD-ROM databases. Either method depends upon the library being accessible (open), the CD-ROM workstations being available, and you having the time to visit. If these conditions are not met, or if you would prefer to search a range of medical databases from the comfort of your own workstation, at a time that is convenient to yourself, you can access these databases, *free of charge*, via the Internet.

In this chapter, I will look at the three most popular medical databases — namely, MEDLINE, the Cochrane Database of Systematic Reviews and EMBASE. Chapter 4 will focus on other useful bibliographic databases including PsychINFO, BIOETHICSLINE and CancerLit.

MEDLINE
http://www.ncbi.nlm.nih.gov/PubMed

MEDLINE, produced by the National Library of Medicine (NLM), is the world's premier biomedical database. Dating from 1966, the MEDLINE database currently contains just under 9 million bibliographic citations drawn from around 3800 biomedical journals. In the current MEDLINE file (the last 5 years) 87% of the citations are to English language sources and 72% have English abstracts.

Free access to MEDLINE, via the Internet, is a relatively new service but one which an ever growing number of Web sites now offer (an annotated list of free MEDLINE sites is available at: http://www.docnet.org.uk/drfelix/). Having looked at several of these services I consider the PubMed MEDLINE, produced by the NLM, to be the best version currently available. The strengths of this service are discussed below:

- Currency of the database. By incorporating data from the Pre-MEDLINE file, citations appear in the database far more quickly than in the traditional versions of MEDLINE. Some measure of the currency of PubMed can be gauged by the observation that articles published in journals such as *JAMA* and *N Engl J Med* are indexed, and thus searchable, within one week of publication; articles from the *BMJ* and *The Lancet* appear within a fortnight of publication.

- Sophisticated searching. By use of pull-down menus it is possible to search specific MEDLINE fields (author name, MeSH term, title word, and so on) and use the Boolean operators (AND, OR and NOT) to combine search terms. PubMed also has a *Clinical Query Filter* that allows you to restrict your search to one of four study categories — therapy, diagnosis, aetiology and prognosis. Once a search has been run and citations have been selected, PubMed also gives you the option to find other related articles.

- Dynamic links with related databases. The NLM is currently establishing links with various publishers to enable MEDLINE searchers to link directly to the full text of a given article. Note, however, that most publishers will require you to set up a credit account before the full text is displayed.

In addition, many MEDLINE articles have links to other related databases. For example, a search of PubMed for references on new variants of CJD highlights, amongst other items, an article by J Collinge[3]. Clicking on the title not only delivers the full citation to your desktop but also enables you to link directly to the relevant part of the *Online Mendelian Inheritance in Man* (OMIM) database where you can find a detailed analysis of CJD (see Figures 3.1 and 3.2). Within OMIM you can then link to other relevant sources including the *Human Gene Mutation Database* at Cardiff University [http://www.uwcm.ac.uk/uwcm/mg/hgmd0.html] and the *Genome Database* at Johns Hopkins University [http://gdbwww.gdb.org/gdb].

Cochrane Database of Systematic Reviews
http://www.hcn.net.au/cochrane/intro.htm

The Cochrane Database of Systematic Reviews (CDSR) is the best single source of reliable evidence about the effects of health care. Concentrating on the results of controlled trials the reviews are highly structured and systematic, with evidence included or excluded on the basis of explicit quality criteria. Although the complete, full-text version of this database is not freely available on the Internet, the Health Communications Network WWW site in

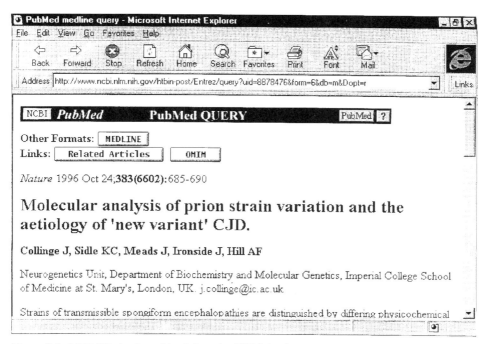

Figure 3.1   MEDLINE citation with a link to the OMIM database

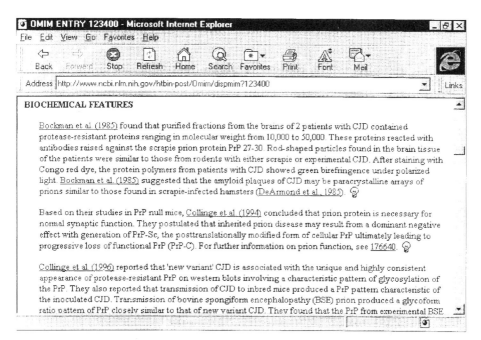

Figure 3.2   The OMIM database, with links back to MEDLINE

Australia provides users with an opportunity to view the detailed abstracts of all the Cochrane reviews published to date (228 reviews as of September 1997).

To facilitate browsing, the reviews are arranged according to the Cochrane Collaborative Review Group headings. Thus, an obstetrician can link directly to reviews carried out by the Neonatal and the Pregnancy and Childbirth groups, whilst an ophthalmologist can concentrate on those reviews performed by the Eyes and Vision Group. The database also clearly indicates whether the reviews are new or have been updated in the past 3 months.

The CDSR provides health professionals with clear and unambiguous evidence-based findings. For example, the review that compares the merits of two instruments used in assisted vaginal delivery concludes, 'the use of vacuum extractor rather than forceps for assisted delivery can be expected to result in substantial reductions in maternal morbidity'[4].

EMBASE
http://www.healthgate.com/HealthGate/price/embase.html

EMBASE, the Excerpta Medica database, is another comprehensive source of biomedical information, including more than 6.5 million records. Though inevitably there is some overlap with MEDLINE, EMBASE is the more comprehensive source for information in pharmacology and psychiatry. EMBASE also indexes a greater number of European and Asian journals than its MEDLINE counterpart.

To help users perform more precise and accurate searches the EMBASE database is split into distinct subject categories. 13 'subsets' currently exist including EMBASE Drugs and Pharmacology, EMBASE Cardiology and EMBASE Paediatrics.

Before you can access these databases you must complete an online registration form at the HealthGate WWW site. Once the registration has been accepted — typically within a few seconds — you will be given unlimited access to search any of the EMBASE subsets and view the titles of any articles, completely free of charge. For every detailed reference you wish to see — author, title, source, and abstract — a fee of $1.50 is levied.

REFERENCES

1   Smith R. What clinical information do doctors need. *BMJ* 1997;**313**:1062–8

2   Wyatt J. Information for clinicians: uses and sources of medical knowledge. *Lancet* 1991;**338**:1368–73

3   Collinge J, Sidle KC, Meads J, Ironside J, Hill AF. Molecular analysis of prion strain variation and the aetiology of 'new variant' CJD. *Nature* 1996;**383**:685–90

4   Johanson RB, Menon VJ. Vacuum extraction vs forceps delivery. [Updated 19th February 1997] *Cochrane Database of Systematic Reviews*. <URL: http://www.hcn.net.au/cochrane/abstracts/ab000166.htm> [Accessed 16 September 1997]

Medical databases on the Internet: part 2

Though the databases MEDLINE, EMBASE and the Cochrane Database of Systematic Reviews (Chapter 3) address the information needs of most health professionals, most of the time, there are occasions when other subject-specific databases need to be searched. This chapter will introduce a number of these databases, all of which can be accessed via the Internet. Unless stated to the contrary, all the resources discussed here are available free of charge.

BIOETHICSLINE
http://www.healthgate.com/HealthGate/MEDLINE/search.shtml

Issues such as xenotransplantation and physician-assisted suicide force all of us to examine the ethical implications of medical research and practice. One database which can be searched to help identify current research, legal judgments and public opinion in matters relating to the ethics of biomedical research and healthcare is BIOETHICSLINE.

Dating from 1973, BIOETHICSLINE provides health professionals with a comprehensive, one-stop source to the world's bioethical literature. For example, searching this database to see what had been published on the topic of 'genetic screening and health insurance' I retrieved a substantial number of references, including newspaper articles, books, and court judgments. Source material of this kind is *not* indexed by MEDLINE.

BIOETHICSLINE also provides users with an opportunity to see how attitudes and opinions change over time. A search for stories about the 'test tube baby' around the time of the birth of Louise Brown yields numerous articles in which the ethics of *in-vitro* fertilization are debated. The same search run against the 1995–1997 BIOETHICSLINE file shows that the ethical debate is now more concerned with the issue of whether or not IVF should be made available to older women.

CancerLit

http://cancernet.nci.nih.gov/canlit/cltopic.htm

CancerLit, a product of the National Cancer Institute (NCI), is a database of references to published journal articles, conference proceedings, government reports, and monographs that relate to cancer.

Recognizing the inherent difficulty in constructing an effective search strategy for cancer information — information overload is the most common problem — the NCI has created 'Topic Searches' which pull together recent articles on frequently requested subjects (see Figure 4.1). Within each topic search — breast cancers, eye cancers, and so on — you can elect to look at references that focus on specific aspects such as chemotherapy, radiotherapy or surgery.

If a defined 'Topic Search' does not meet your needs the entire CancerLit database of 1.3 million citations, dating from 1963, can be searched at: http://cnetdb.nci.nih.gov/cancerlit.shtml

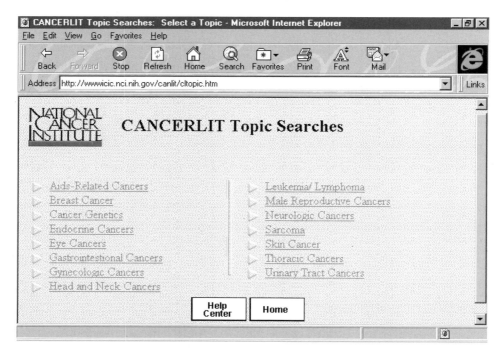

Figure 4.1 **CANCERLIT topic searches**

PsycINFO

http://www.healthgate.com/HealthGate/price/b.psycinfo.html

If your information requirements relate more to psychology, or the psychological aspects of medicine, the PsycINFO database produced by the American Psychological Association is an excellent resource. Coverage spans 1967 to the present, and includes international material selected from more than 1300 periodicals written in over 25 languages.

When researching this column I searched the PsycINFO database to see if anything had been written on the psychological consequences of using the Internet. Inevitably there were a number of articles that discussed 'cybersex' and how sexually explicit expression on the Internet can be regulated. More alarmingly, there is a growing literature on the addictive nature of the Internet (see Figure 4.2)

As with BIOETHICSLINE, the unique collection of source material in PsycINFO ensures that your search will always find material different from that identified by MEDLINE.

Before you can search the PsycINFO database you must complete an online registration form at the HealthGate WWW site. You can then search the database and view the titles of any

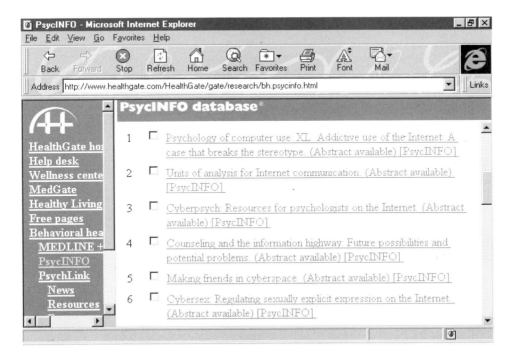

Figure 4.2 **A search of PsycINFO for articles about the psychological consequences of using the Internet**

articles, completely free of charge. For every *detailed* reference you wish to see — author, title, source, and abstract — a fee of £0.75 is levied.

WISDOM — Sources of Biomedical Research Funding
http://wisdom.wellcome.ac.uk/wisdom/fundhome.html

At some time or another most health professionals seek funding to support some biomedical research they wish to undertake. Identifying appropriate funders, however, has always been a time-consuming process as candidates manually sift the numerous grants directories such as the *Awards Almanac, Grants Register* and the *Educational Grants Directory*[1–3]. One Internet product that can greatly simplify this process is the WISDOM: Sources of Biomedical Research Funding Database, produced by the Wellcome Trust. This database contains descriptions of 400 funding schemes offered by 100 UK organizations supporting biomedical research. Information includes the type and purpose of the award, the amount of funding available and the full application procedure, including contact details. It also provides background information on funding policy, total annual expenditure on biomedical research and publications for each funding body.

Using WISDOM a doctor interested in undertaking research into some aspect of rheumatism for example, will quickly find that the organizations most likely to fund this include the Arthritis and Rheumatism Council for Research, the Nuffield Foundation and the National Back Pain Association.

Though *some* of the organizations in the WISDOM database do offer grants for research projects outside of the UK, its focus is most definitely on UK-based research. If you seek an award to undertake research outside of the UK, the GrantsNet database — developed by the Howard Hughes Medical Institute in collaboration with the American Association for the Advancement of Science is worth looking at. To search this database point your Web browser at: http://www.grantsnet.org/

OTHER DATABASES — IN BRIEF

Database of Abstracts of Reviews of Effectiveness (DARE)
http://nhscrd.york.ac.uk

For high-quality research reviews that look at the *effectiveness* of health care interventions and the management and organization of health services, DARE, produced by the NHS Centre for Reviews and Dissemination at York University, is recommended.

Pharmaceutical Information Network (PharmInfoNet)

http://pharminfo.com/

Provided by VirSci Corporation, PharmInfoNet provides high-quality *independent* assessments of therapeutics and advances in new drug development A search of the drugs database (by generic or trade name) leads you to a series of full-text articles published in *Medical Sciences Bulletin*. A search for sumatriptan highlighted several papers including 'Sumatriptan for migraine' and 'Sumatriptan: is Chest Pain Esophageal in Origin'?

AIDSLINE, AIDSDRUGS & AIDSTRIALS

http://www.healthgate.com/choice/AMA/search.html

For information about AIDS these three databases produced by the National Library of Medicine should be consulted.

REFERENCES

1   Ferrara MH, Jaszczak, eds. *The Awards Almanac: an International Guide to Career, Research and Education Funds.* London: St James Press, 1996

2   Austin R, ed. *The Grants Register, 1998: the Complete Guide to Postgraduate Funding Worldwide. 16th edn.* Basingstoke: Macmillan Reference

3   Smyth J, Wallace K, eds. *The Educational Grants Directory, 1996/97 edition.* London: Directory of Social Change, 1996

Internet discussion lists

The principal reason why people seek Internet connectivity is the desire to communicate electronically with friends and colleagues. Though much of this electronic communication takes place one-to-one, it is equally easy to communicate with hundreds (or thousands) of users who have a common interest. This chapter will explain the mechanics of an Internet discussion list — how you join a list and send messages — as well as highlighting practical issues such as how you can find lists relevant to your specialty and how you can minimize the time spent reading irrelevant postings. In true Internet style this piece will take the form of an FAQ document (frequently asked questions).

WHAT IS A DISCUSSION LIST?

Discussion lists (or mailing lists) are subject-specific groups that are participated in and distributed by e-mail. Once you have joined a list — for example *sports-med*, a list created to discuss all aspects of sports medicine — every message that is posted to this list is copied to your electronic mailbox. As this task of copying and forwarding mail messages to every list member is performed by a computer software program, the effort for the individual is the same as sending an e-mail to a single colleague. No charges are levied to 'subscribe' to any discussion list.

Discussion lists are an excellent way for health professionals to solicit opinion, air concerns and discuss matters of mutual interest. For example, subscribers to the *GP-UK* discussion list recently discussed the NHS network, the efficacy of troglitizone, and whether an eight minute appointment slot is long enough for an effective consultation. As each mail message is sent to the 600+ subscribers, most postings generate some response and discussion.

CAN ANYONE JOIN ANY LIST?

Every discussion list has its own set of rules governing issues such as who can join and post messages, and whether or not postings have to be vetted (moderated) by the list owner. Thus, the list *Surginet*, established to facilitate discussion on all aspects of general surgery, is only open to those who can demonstrate their 'medical credentials', whilst postings to the cystic fibrosis list, *cystic-l*, are open to anyone. Moderated lists tend to be less active than open ones, though the level of discussion is usually of far higher quality.

HOW DO I FIND LISTS RELEVANT TO MY INTERESTS?

With recent estimates suggesting that the number of Internet discussion lists now exceeds 85 000 the greatest problem facing any Internet user is in identifying relevant lists. In part this problem can be addressed by searching the *Directory of Mailing Lists Database* at http://www.liszt.com (See Figure 5.1).

As an example of the range of lists available, a search for 'arthritis' identified five potentially relevant discussion forums including *arthritis-l*, a general discussion forum about arthritis, and *OMERACT*, a tightly defined list that looks exclusively at outcome measures in rheumatoid arthritis clinical trials. The Liszt database also provides additional

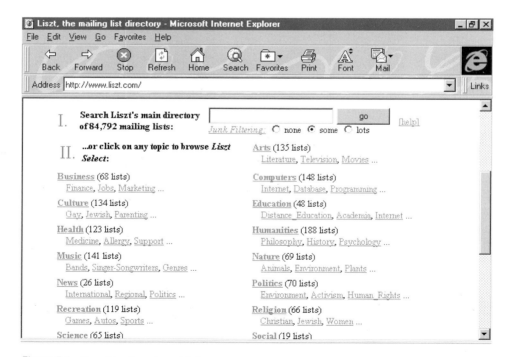

Figure 5.1 **Searching for relevant lists**

information about each list including the average number of postings, and whether the list is open or closed. If this information is unavailable instruction is provided on how to obtain it.

Though the coverage of the Liszt database is extensive, it does not index the 1800 discussion lists hosted by Mailbase. Since these lists originate in the UK and are only established if they can be seen to benefit higher education and research communities, they are particularly useful to health professionals practising in the UK. Names and descriptions of Mailbase lists can be searched at http://www.mailbase.ac.uk/search.html. A search of this database for discussion forums that may be of interest to a geneticist identified thirteen lists including *psych-genetic*, which concerns itself with psychological issues surrounding genetic screening, and *inborn-errors*, set up to disseminate research into inherited metabolic diseases.

HOW DO I JOIN AND CONTRIBUTE TO A DISCUSSION LIST?

Though it may sound trivial, one of the most important things you need to understand about discussion lists is the difference between the address of the mailing list and the address of the listserver. Messages that relate to the administration of the list (joining, leaving and so on) must be sent to the listserver, whilst contributions to the discussion should be sent directly to the list. Failure to comply with this protocol results in 'unsubscribe' postings being distributed to every subscriber.

If you want to join the discussion list *psych-genetic* your message to the listserver should be as follows:

    To: mailbase@mailbase.ac.uk

    Subject: leave blank

    Message: subscribe psych-genetic *firstname surname*

To contribute to the discussion list *psych-genetic*, your message might be:

    To: psych-genetic@mailbase.ac.uk

    Subject: Xenotransplantation seminar

    Message: Professionals concerned about the ethics of substituting animals organs . . .

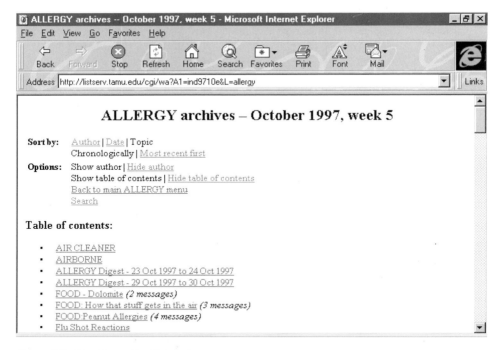

Figure 5.2 **The Allergy List Web archive**

HOW I CAN USE DISCUSSION LISTS EFFECTIVELY?

Though discussion lists can be very informative and entertaining they can also be very time consuming. Though the 96 messages posted to the list *evidence-based health* in an average month may be manageable, the 528 messages posted to *GP-UK* may be more problematic. You only have to forget to empty your e-mail box for a couple of days to appreciate the difficulties posed by high-volume discussion lists.

This difficulty can be overcome if the list maintains a hypertext Web archive of all postings. For example, the Allergy List has a Web archive which anyone can access [http:// listserv.tamu.edu/archives/allergy.html] This site not only allows you to read all messages sent to this list — at a time and frequency you can dictate — but also provides readers with the opportunity to keyword search the postings. Moreover, in a move which I hope will be adopted by other sites hosting hypertext Web archives, the Allergy site also produces a 'table of contents' to each week's postings. This feature ensures that you only need read those postings which truly interest you (see Figure 5.2). Web-based archives also enable you to assess the relevance of a list before you commit yourself to a subscription. If a discussion list does not support a Web-based archive then it is important to read its 'info' file, which will describe its purpose, scope and intended audience. Also, if a list strays from its original objectives, alert the list owner. If the list continues to generate irrelevant postings, use your right to unsubscribe.

Evidence-based medicine on the Internet

Whatever the long-term outcomes of practising evidence-based medicine prove to be for the delivery of effective health care, there is little doubt of the impact it has had on the printing and publishing industries. For example, in the past 12 months the MEDLINE database alone has indexed more than 300 articles on this topic. Over the same period, a search of *Whitaker's Books in Print* for titles that contain the words 'evidence based' identifies more than a dozen new books, whilst *Ulrich's Periodicals Directory* records the launch of five new journals on this theme. Fear of information overload is compounded by the results of an Internet search which highlights the existence of 5000+ evidence-based medicine Web sites.

The purpose of this chapter is to highlight a few resources on the Internet that can help the busy health professional understand and practise evidence-based medicine.

EBM at McMaster University
http://hiru.hirunet.mcmaster.ca/ebm/default.htm

McMaster University in Canada is generally regarded as the home of the evidence-based medicine (EBM) movement. Not surprisingly, therefore, the Web site at this institution is an excellent first stop in your trawl for relevant information. Beginning with an overview, visitors to this Web resource are presented with a clear definition of EBM and details of how McMaster is building a residency programme in which a key goal is to 'practice, role-model, teach, and help residents become highly adept' in this new way of practising medicine.

Central to the practice of EBM is the need for clinicians critically to appraise the information they find. At the McMaster Web site this skill is taught through a number of *Users' Guides* that explain how you can use the medical literature to resolve a treatment decision. For example, the guide entitled *How to Use an Article about Therapy or Prevention* stresses the need to ask yourself questions such as 'are the results of the study valid?', 'was the clinical trial randomized?', 'were the groups treated equally?', and 'will the results help me in caring for my patients?'. Any danger that the discussion may become too theoretical is minimized by frequent reference to real clinical studies. Thus, if you question the importance of using evidence from *randomized* clinical trials to support a clinical decision, you will be reminded of the various randomized trials that *contradicted* the results of less rigorous trials. These include the findings that steroids may increase (rather than reduce) mortality in patients with sepsis and that plasmapheresis does not benefit patients with polymyositis.

Emphasizing again the view that EBM is a practical subject and one which should be used in the day-to-day clinical environment the McMaster site provides links to various EBM tools that are available on the Internet. Included here is the Obstetric and Gynaecology Toolbox (http://www.cpmc.columbia.edu/resources/obgyntools/) which, amongst other things, allows you to conduct an obstetrical ultrasound analysis to calculate estimated gestational ages and fetal weights based on various measurements (Figure 6.1), and the Heart Attack Survival Calculator (http://www.mediqual.com/library/amicalc/heart.htm) where values are entered to determine the probability of survival (Figure 6.2).

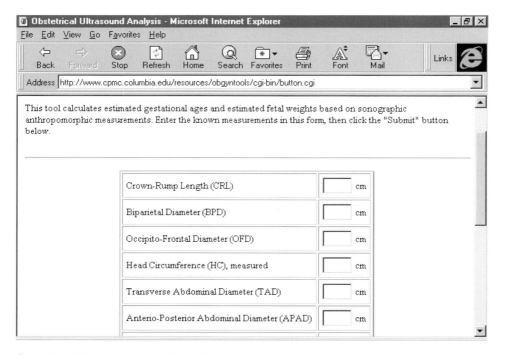

Figure 6.1　**Obstetric ultrasound analysis**

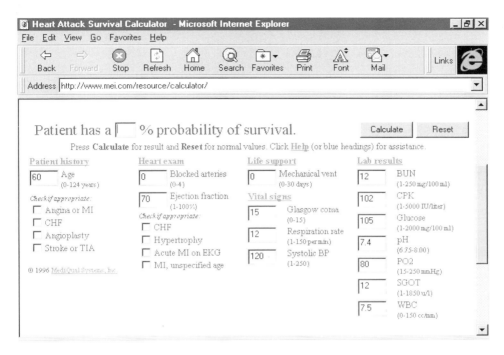

Figure 6.2 **Heart attack survival calculator**

Turning Research into Practice (TRIP)

http://www.gwent.nhs.gov.uk/trip/test-search.html

One of the difficulties facing clinicians who wish to practise EBM is the disparate way research findings are disseminated. Though the Cochrane Database (http://www.cochrane.co.uk/abstracts) is the premier source for identifying results of systematic reviews, other sources such as clinical practice guidelines and briefing papers may also be of interest. In recognition of this the Primary Care Clinical Effectiveness Team for Gwent have created the TRIP database which provides a single searchable index to 14 EBM resources thus providing a one-stop link to over 1150 evidence-based topics. Sources indexed by TRIP include the Cochrane Database, the Canadian Clinical Practice Guidelines Infobase, and the evidence-based healthcare journal *Bandolier*.

Searching this database to find evidence and best practice for the care of patients with prostate cancer I was pointed to ten relevant studies including the 'Prostate Cancer Review' published in *Bandolier*, the NHS Centre for Reviews and Dissemination *Effectiveness Matters Bulletin* on 'Screening for prostate cancer' and the POEMS (Patient Oriented Evidence that Matters) resource 'Conservative treatment of prostate cancer' (Figure 6.3).

33

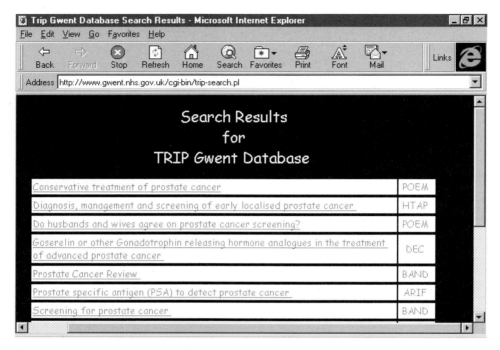

Figure 6.3 **The TRIP database—results of a search on prostate cancer**

Health Services Technology Assessment Text (HSTAT)

http://text.nlm.nih.gov/

A similar resource to TRIP, though one with an exclusive emphasis on US resources, is the Health Services Technology Assessment Text database. This resource enables the clinician to search several full-text databases simultaneously, including the *Evidence Reports* from the Agency for Health Care Policy and Research (AHCPR), the NIH *Consensus Development Reports and Statements* and the Public Health Services *Guide to Clinical Preventive Services.* When I searched this database for publications on cystic fibrosis, the resources included an *NIH Consensus Statement* entitled 'Genetic testing for cystic fibrosis' and an AHCPR Technology Assessment report on 'Single and double lung transplantation'.

Medical journals on the World Wide Web

Tucked away in a recent issue of the *Washington Post* was a news item that could have major implications for the medical publishing industry: a Washington Publisher, National Academy Press, had increased its sales by 17% in the year after its decision to post, in full text, 1700 of its current titles on the World Wide Web[1]. Anyone with Internet access can read any of these titles completely free of charge[2].

Though many publishers — especially those with a more commercial agenda — may not be quite ready to make this quantum leap forward, most have made a move in this direction and have established some sort of Web presence. Some 2680 medical and life science journals already have their own Web sites[3]. In this article I discuss some features of electronic journals as well as provide details of the most popular and influential medical journals that can now be accessed via the Internet.

ELECTRONIC JOURNALS

Internet services develop and evolve with extraordinary speed, and this 'tradition of change' has been mirrored by various journal Web sites. Writing in May 1995, on the launch of the *BMJ* Web site, the editor remarked that from now on 'users will now be able to scan the list of contents, read the editor's choice, and download full structured abstracts. Some articles will be available in full text'[4]. By December 1997 this vision had developed to one where, from March 1998, Internet users will be able to see the *entire* journal in full text, receive each week's table of contents by e-mail and receive a customized alerting service of new articles on defined topics[5]. Access to the *BMJ* site will continue to be free.

In addition to providing an electronic version of a paper journal, some Web sites have been quick to exploit opportunities offered by the Internet. For example, the *Journal of Clinical Investigation* provides hypertext links, from every article, to the PubMed MEDLINE service. This feature allows the reader to search for other articles by the same author, or identify other papers on a related topic (see Figure 7.1).

Similarly, recognizing the ease by which Internet users can communicate (e-mail) the *Medical Journal of Australia* is using its Web site to develop a new model for peer review[6]. Articles submitted for publication are posted on the *MJA* Web site along with an invitation for readers to e-mail the editor with their views and comments. Open scrutiny of the peer review process is established since every review, along with the author's response, is posted on the Web site.

SIX OF THE BEST

To help readers find the Web sites of some of the most popular journals I have compiled a *Six of the Best — Quick Reference Guide*. In compiling this guide I discounted either circulation figures or rankings based on impact factors. The former method promotes 'association journals' at the expense of subscription titles such as *The Lancet*, whilst the impact rankings[7] put titles used by researchers — such as *Cell* and the *Annual Review of Immunology* — higher than those used by physicians in clinical practice. Lacking any suitable scientific criteria, I base my *Six of the Best* on my observations, as a medical librarian, of what

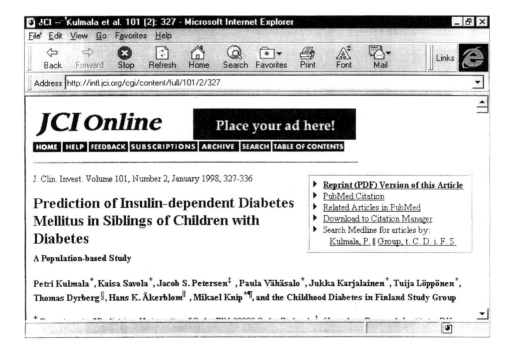

Figure 7.1 **Journal of Clinical Investigation** online: options to link to PubMed and view article in PDF format

general non-specialty journals physicians read and scan. All the titles cited here can be accessed free of charge. 'ToC by email?' refers to whether or not the Web site offers an electronic table of contents service.

Title:	*Annals of Internal Medicine*
Web address:	htp://www.acponline.org/journals/annals/annaltoc.htm
Contents pages:	Available from January 1996
ToC by e-mail?	No
Full text:	Several original articles are available in full-text format, along with the editorials, letters and update columns
Comments:	The Web site also has a powerful search engine that enables you to search for articles published in the *Annals*

Title:	*British Medical Journal*
Web address:	htp://www.bmj.com
Contents pages:	Online from January 1997 [by the end of 1998, six years of data will be available]
ToC by e-mail?	Yes
Full text:	The entire journal, from January 1997, is available in full text. Moreover, the Web site also contains supplemental data which the paper version does not carry, due to space restrictions. For example, the Web version of the article by McColl *et al.*[8], on GP's perceptions of evidence-based medicine, contains a copy of the questionnaire the authors used to collect their data
Comments:	The site also has special collections that bring together articles on topics such as BSE–CJD as well as full text copies of *BMJ* books including *Statistics at Square 1* and *How to Read a Paper: the Basis of Evidence Based Medicine*

Title:	*JAMA*
Web address:	http://www.ama-assn.org/public/journals/jama/jamahome.htm
Contents pages:	Online from July 1995
ToC by e-mail?	No
Full text:	Some original contributions from each issue are available in full text. Those which are not in full-text format have detailed online abstracts
Comments:	The AMA has also established *JAMA* condition-specific Web sites. These contain a peer reviewed collection of resources on topics including HIV/ AIDS, asthma and migraine

Title:	*Journal of Clinical Investigation*
Web address:	http://intl.jci.org/
Contents pages:	Online archive dating from January 1996
ToC by e-mail?	Yes
Full text:	**All** articles are available in full text. Articles can be read on a standard Web page or as a PDF (portable document format) file. The PDF version enables you to see and print the article as it appears in the paper journal with original page numbering, text layout and fonts
Comments:	Each *JCI* article has dynamic, hypertext links to the MEDLINE database, and articles can be downloaded directly into citation management software. The site also supports a powerful search feature that allows you to search the full text of the *JCI*, and if required, other titles (such as *Blood*, *Pediatrics*, and *Science*) hosted on this Web server

Title:	*The Lancet*
Web address:	http//www.thelancet.com/
Contents pages:	Available online since June 1996
ToC by e-mail?	No
Full text:	The editorials and news items are available in full text. Around 50% of the research articles have online abstracts with hypertext links to the appropriate commentary section. Full text of the entire journal is available to subscribers
Comments:	The *Lancet* site has a searchable appointments database — with 35 vacancies in January 1998 — and details of the forthcoming *Lancet* Conference 'The Challenge of Stroke'. To use the *Lancet* Web site you need to complete an online registration form

Title:	*New England Journal of Medicine*
Web address:	http://www.nejm.org/
Contents pages:	Online archive dating from January 1993
ToC by e-mail?	Yes
Full text:	All editorials, letters, and book reviews are available in full text. All original and review articles have detailed online abstracts with hypertext links that enable you to order a copy of an article. Articles can be faxed or mailed to you at a cost of $10 per item. Subscribers to the print version can access the complete text of the *NEJM* for all issues from January 1993 without incurring any additional charges
Comments:	The *NEJM* site has a number of 'Collections' that contain the full text of selected articles published in this journal. Collections currently available include asthma, breast cancer and kidney diseases

REFERENCES

1   Berselli, B. Read it and weep: online publishing actually boosts sales. *Washington Post* 30 September 1997 [Financial Section] col. 1

2   <URL: http://www.nap.edu/> [Accessed 9 January 1998]

3   Tonosaki M. Effective use of scientific journals' content, abstract, and full text information on the Internet in the fields of medical and life sciences — with their URL addresses. *Online Kensaku*, 1996;**17**(3/4):91–225 <URL: http://omni-ac.uk/mirror/tonoej12.pdf> [Accessed 10 January 1998]

4   Delamothe T. *BMJ* on the Internet. *BMJ* 1994;**310**:1343–344<URL: http://www.bmj.com.archive/6991e-1.htm. [Accessed 12 January 1998]

5   Delamothe T. Developing www.bmj.com. *BMJ* 1997;**315**:1558 <URL: http://www.bmj.com/archive/7122/7122e5.htm> [Accessed 12 January 1998]

6   <URL: http://www.mja.com.au/public/papers/papers.htm> [Accessed 13 January 1998]

7   Institute for Scientific Information, Journal performance indicators: impact rankings — Science Citation Index Philadelphia: ISI, 1997

8   McColl A, *et al.* General Practitioners' perceptions of the route to evidence based medicine: a questionnaire survey. *BMJ* 1998;**316**:361–5 <URL: http://www.bmj.com/cgi/content/full/316/7128/361> [Accessed 21 August 1998]

Consumer health information on the Internet

The White Paper *The new NHS: A Modern Dependable*[1] promotes the vision that the National Health Service must provide patients with more and better information about health, illness and the Service. The Internet—along with public access media such as digital TV—is identified as a medium through which this information will be delivered. Evidence already exists that consumers are using the Internet to find health information. One report, by FIND-SVP, concluded that 36% of US citizens who can access the Internet use it to find health and medical information[2]. More anecdotally, we hear of patients who turn up at the surgery armed with printouts from the Internet. To provide a brief guide to consumer health information on the Internet this article highlights some authoritative consumer sites that can be used to answer a range of frequently asked questions.

SELF-HELP GROUPS

Charities Aid Foundation (UK)
http://www.charitynet.org/main.html

Contact-a-Family (UK)
http://www.cafamily.org.uk/

National Organization for Rare Diseases (US)
http://www.rarediseases.org/

Many studies have demonstrated the value of encouraging patients and their relatives to participate in self-help groups[3,4]. One, looking at ovarian cancer support groups, concluded that because of the low rate of cure and high rate of relapse 'psychological interventions to support patients emotionally and to enhance their quality of life should be considered an important complement to medical care'[5].

A good way for clinicians to identify relevant self-help groups is to search the Charities Aid Foundation Web site. Though this site contains details of all kinds of charities—over 90 000

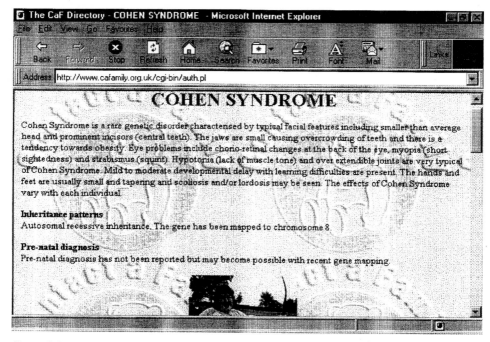

Figure 8.1 **Description of Cohen syndrome from the Contact-a-Family database**

voluntary organizations are listed here — the search facility enables you to focus your enquiry. A search for 'miscarriage' identifies nine self-help groups including the Miscarriage Association (and its various branches) and the Society for Counselling and Information on Miscarriage. If you follow any of these links you will be presented with full contact details of that association, and if available, a hypertext link to its Web site.

For clinicians who have to inform parents that their child has a special need or disability, the Contact-a-Family Web site may prove an invaluable resource (Figure 8.1). This site provides information on numerous medical conditions and syndromes that affect children, along with contact details of family support networks. All the information is clear and unambiguous, and is formatted in a way that makes it ideal for printing out and passing on to parents. A small fee is levied. (See http://www.cafamily.org.uk/form.html for details.)

For details of US and Canadian self-help groups the National Organisation for Rare Diseases (NORD) Web site can be searched. The NORD database contains entries on over 1100 rare disorders, with links to supporting organizations.

PATIENT LEAFLETS

http://www.hebs.scot.nhs.uk/

http://www.healthtouch.com/level1/hi_toc.htm

Information and instructions given to the patient in the surgery or outpatients department can often be reinforced by a printed leaflet. A study published in the *British Journal of General Practice*[6] concluded that providing leaflets to women about the contraceptive pill increases their knowledge of the subject, which in turn could lead to reduction in the number of unplanned pregnancies. Keeping a stock of up-to-date leaflets on a range of subjects can be both time-consuming and expensive in space; both these drawbacks are overcome by using Web-based resources.

The Scottish Health Education Board Web site has several leaflets, mainly covering the Health of the Nation target areas, which are suitable for patients. For example, the pages dealing with mental health have information on topics such as eating disorders, schizophrenia and stress, whilst the heart disease section has a 'hassle free food guide' which provides hints on how to make meals that are enjoyable, easy and healthy.

For more disease-specific information leaflets the Health Touch Web site is worth visiting. The information here is derived exclusively from professional organizations and presented in a format appropriate for printing and distribution. Each document states when it was last revised. A search for 'osteoporosis', for example, identifies several leaflets, including *What is Osteoporosis?* authored by the American College of Rheumatology and *Women and Osteoporosis* written by Women's Health Initiative.

DRUG INFORMATION

http://www.intelihealth.com/

A study on patients' use of prescribed medicines concluded that provision of 'relevant information in a clear and concise manner' would improve compliance[7]. Earlier work had shown that up to 50% of what the doctor tells the patient is immediately forgotten[8], so there is a good argument for providing the information in a written format which the patient can take away.

The US Pharmacopeia provides patients with accurate and authoritative drug information in a clear and jargon-free format. Visitors to this site have the option of either searching the database (by trade or generic name) or browsing through an alphabetic listing of drugs. Once a drug has been selected from the database the information presented is in three parts — general advice for the patient, patient education leaflets that describe the use and side-effects

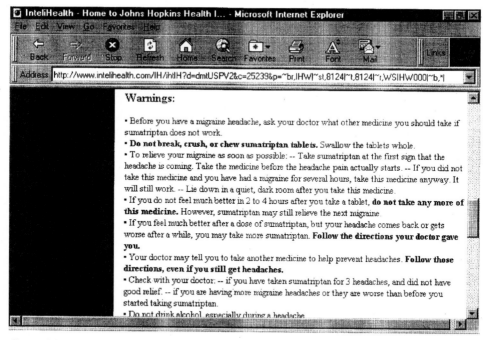

Figure 8.2 **US Pharmacopeia advice about sumatriptan**

of this type of drug, and medicine charts that show the dosage variations with images of the various pills.

For example, the migraine sufferer who has been prescribed sumatriptan is informed that the drug should be taken 'at the first sign that the headache is coming...but if you do not feel much better in 2 to 4 hours after a tablet is taken, do **not** take any more of this medicine for the same migraine' (Figure 8.2). Instruction is also provided on how the tablets should be taken — 'do not break, crush, or chew the tablets before swallowing them' — and all known side-effects are clearly listed. From a patient's perspective one of the very useful aspects of this source is the way in which the adverse effects are divided into those which require 'immediate medical attention' and those that 'usually do not require medical attention'.

Information in the US Pharmacopeia is derived from a peer-review consensus process that involves medical specialty and professional practice advisory panels.

REFERENCES

1   *The New NHS: A Modern Dependable* (Cm 3807) London: HMSO, 1997

2   Brown MS. Consumer health and medical information on the Internet: supply and demand. FIBD-SVP Inc. 1997 <URL: http://erg.findsvp.com/health/mktginfo.html> [Accessed 8 February 1998]

3   Montazeri A. A descriptive study of a cancer support group. *Eur J Cancer Care* 1996;**5**:32–37

4   Guidry JJ, Aday LA, Zhang D, Winn RJ. The role of informal and formal social support networks for patients with cancer. *Cancer Pract* 1997;**5**:241–46

5   Sivesind DM, Baile WF. An ovarian cancer support group *Cancer Pract* 1997;**5**:247–51

6   Smith LF, Whitfield MJ. Women's knowledge of taking oral contraceptive pills correctly and of emergency contraception: effects of providing information leaflets in general practice. *Br J Gen Practice* 1995;**45**:409–14

7   Griffith S. A review of the factors associated with patient compliance and the taking of prescribed medicines. *Br J Gen Practice* 1990;**40**:114–16

8   Lee P. Memory for medical information. *Br J Soc Clin Psychol* 1979;**18**:245–55

Health statistics on the World Wide Web

Writing in the *BMJ*, O'Dowd[1] used the term 'heartsink' to describe patients who exasperate, defeat and overwhelm their doctors by their behaviour. If librarians classified their clients in this fashion the reader who requested statistical data on the prevalence of a particular disease might find himself similarly labelled. Up-to-date health statistics have always proved difficult to find, and even when relevant sources have been unearthed the data are rarely in the format required.

With the development of the Web—and the resultant information explosion—health statistics from numerous countries are only a mouse-click away. This paper will highlight some key sources on the Internet.

VITAL STATISTICS

National Center for Health Statistics (US)
http://www.cdc.gov/nchswww

Office of National Statistics (UK)
http://www.ons.gov.uk/

WHO Health Report 1997 (World)
http://www.who.ch/whr/1997/whr-e.htm

For statistical information relating to the UK, the Web site of the Office of National Statistics is a useful resource. Its 'Population and Vital Statistics' pages provide information on the make-up of the UK population—size of ethnic minorities, percentage of the population over retirement age and so on—and other key data elements such as infant mortality and the number of legal abortions. When available, comparable figures for selected years back to 1974 are cited.

Readers seeking health statistics from the USA should visit the National Center for Health Statistics Web site. Arranging the data by broad subject categories—birth, infertility, surgical procedures — the visitor can quickly navigate to the appropriate Web page. Specific questions can then be posed and answered. For example, in the section headed 'death' you can identify the leading causes of death and the latest infant mortality figures. Although the data are presented in summary format, the original source (with supporting data) is available via a hypertext link.

For a more global perspective on health, the 'Fifty Facts' from the 1997 WHO Health Report can be consulted. Key statistics from this source include the size of the world's population — currently standing at 5.8 billion — and the finding that 33% of all deaths in 1996 were due to infectious or parasitic diseases.

DISEASE-SPECIFIC STATISTICS

Cancer

International Agency for Research in Cancer
http://www-dep.iarc.fr/dataava/dataicon.htm

The Cancer Mondial Web site, produced by IARC, has a database of cancer statistics which can be interrogated by data type (incidence/mortality), by type of cancer and by country. From this *single* site you can obtain statistical data on 28 types of cancer from 95 different countries. (See Figure 9.1.)

Heart disease and stroke

American Heart Association
http://www.amhrt.org

Coronary Prevention Group
http://healthpro.org.uk

Cardiovascular diseases are responsible for around 20% of deaths world-wide and are the principal cause of death in developed countries. Both the American Heart Association and the UK Coronary Prevention Group publish a range of 'factsheets' that provide a digest of statistics relating to cardiovascular diseases. Particularly useful are the AHA Biostatistical pages where data are grouped according to specific populations (African-Americans, women, for example) and risk factors.

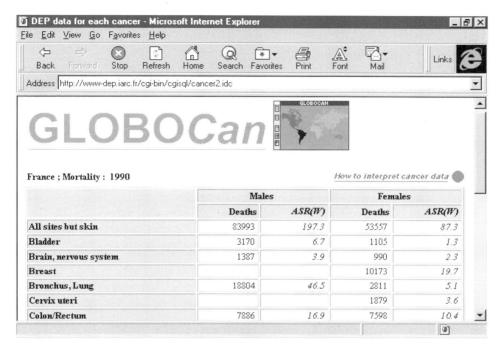

Figure 9.1 **GLOBOCan: cancer mortality statistics; France**

AIDS and sexual health

United Nations
http://www.unaids.org/highband/fact/index.html

The United Nations AIDS Web site has a wealth of statistical information on the prevalence of HIV/AIDS throughout the world. Key documents here include the 1997 report on the 'Global HIV/AIDS Epidemic' which details the numbers of people infected, new infections and deaths, and the 1996 'HIV/AIDS Epidemiology in sub-Saharan Africa'.

Creutzfeldt–Jakob disease

UK CJD Surveillance Unit
http://www.cjd.ed.ac.uk/

The UK Creutzfeldt–Jakob Disease Surveillance Unit provides figures for the number of confirmed cases of the new variant of CJD and referrals of suspected cases of CJD. The Web site also provides data on the incidence of CJD across Europe.

49

Other diseases

When searching the Internet to identify statistical information about other diseases — say, the prevalence of asthma — you are more likely to find the answer if you *first* consider which body or organization is likely to publish this type of information. In the case of asthma, organizations such as the National Institute of Allergy and Infectious Diseases and the National Asthma Campaign would be worth contacting. On visiting the Web site of these organizations I was able to find the 'National Asthma Audit 97/98'[2], which highlighted the latest data on the prevalence, cost and impact of asthma in the UK, and the NIAID fact sheet entitled 'Asthma and Allergy Statistics'[3].

If a search proves unsuccessful, the WHO Statistical Information System (WHOSIS) Web site (http://www.who.ch/whosis) or the Epidemiology section of the World Wide Web Virtual Library (http://www.epibiostat.ucsf.edu/epidem/epidem.html) may provide some useful leads.

EPIDEMIOLOGICAL JOURNALS

Morbidity & Mortality Weekly Report
http://www.cdc.gov/epo/mmwr/mmwr.html

Weekly Epidemiological Report
http://www.who.ch/wer/

Communicable Disease Prevention & Control
http://www.cdpc.com

For the very latest information about the incidence of various diseases the weekly epidemiological newsletters published by the WHO and the CDC are particularly useful, and are freely available on the Internet. If these sources prove too detailed, a useful digest, augmented with communicable disease reports from countries such as the UK, Canada and Australia, can be accessed at the Communicable Disease Prevention & Control Web site.

REFERENCES

1. O'Dowd TC. Five years of heartsink patients in general practice. *BMJ* **297**:528–30

2. <URL: http://www.asthma.org.uk/Pressreleases/mainprd.htm>
    [Accessed 1 March 1998]

3. <URL: http://www.niaid.nih.gov/factsheets/allergystat.htm>
    [Accessed 1 March 1998]

Medical education on the World Wide Web

Some five years after the release of Mosaic, the first graphical Web browser, there are clear signs that the Web is growing up and becoming an integral part of our lives. In the commercial sector this maturity is reflected in online shopping and banking, whereas in health we have seen the development of Web versions of MEDLINE, and electronic journals. Perhaps the clearest indication that the Web has come of age was seen when the National Cancer Institute published exclusively on its Web site the findings relating to prevention of breast cancer by tamoxifen[1].

In parallel with these developments there has been a concerted move by several organizations to deliver medical education over the Web. Though some of these services can be very informal — such as providing a current awareness alerting service — others allow health professionals to prepare for examinations and earn continuing medical education (CME) credits. This article will highlight some of the Web-based educational initiatives that can be pursued at a time and location of one's own choosing.

ONLINE CME

NIH Consensus Development Program
http://text.nlm.nih.gov/nih/upload-v3/Continuing__Education/cme.html

Medscape–CME
http://www.medscape.com/

One of the more common ways CME is delivered over the Web is in the form of online examinations, with CME credits awarded to those who pass.

At the National Institutes of Health (NIH) Web site it is possible to study for and take an online examination based on NIH Consensus Statements and Technology Assessments. Topics available for study include 'Ovarian cancer: screening, treatment and follow-up', 'Management of hepatitis C' and the 'Treatment of chronic pain and insomnia'. For each topic, students are required to read the relevant NIH statement and then complete a multiple-choice questionnaire. This is submitted electronically and the score is immediately calculated. Students who achieve a score of 70% or more receive a certificate for 1 hour of CME. These courses have been accredited by the Accreditation Council for CME, and NIH does not charge for the examinations.

The small number of CME topics at the NIH Web site is in stark contrast to that offered by Medscape. With more than 200 CME accredited articles the team at Medscape have devised a 'CME Locator' to help users find articles on a defined topic. To earn a CME credit, students are obliged to read three articles and submit written commentary, of 50 words or more, on each one. Unlike the NIH CME pages, most of the CME activities at Medscape are fee-based.

Though none of the CME credits earned at the NIH or Medscape Web sites can be 'cashed' in the UK, the educational value of these sites is still considerable.

MEMBERSHIP AND FELLOWSHIP EXAMINATIONS

MRCP Part 1 Question Bank
http://homepages.enterprise.net/djenkins/mcqs/

X-ray Files
http://www-ipg.umds.ac.uk/~acd/xrayfiles/index.htm

Doctors preparing for Membership and Fellowship Examinations of the Royal Colleges will find much useful information at the awarding bodies' Web site[2]. Absent from these pages, however, are any past examination papers, which could help candidates prepare more effectively.

One unofficial site that goes some way in addressing this issue is the MRCP Part 1 question bank created by Dr Dean Jenkins, specialist registrar at Llandough Hospital, Cardiff. It consists of 900 questions of the type seen in the MRCP Part 1 examination and students can either work through the entire collection or run a search against the databank to identify questions on a particular subject. The answer to each question, along with explanatory comments, is revealed by mouse-clicking the 'answer' box (Figure 10.1).

Similarly, students preparing for Part 1 of the Fellowship of the Royal College of Radiologists (FRCR) will find the X-ray File Web site particularly useful. A mix of multiple choice questions and radiological case studies, this site, created and maintained by Dr Andrew Downie of UMDS Guy's and St Thomas' Hospitals, is an excellent example of how the Web can be used to deliver medical education. Those who have advanced

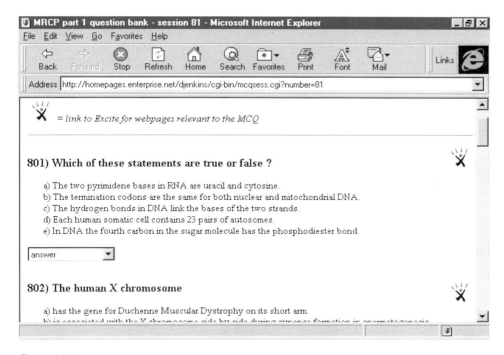

Figure 10.1 **Part of the MRCP part 1 Question Bank**

beyond Part I of the FRCR can turn to the more complex tutorials and case studies (Figure 10.2).

INTERACTIVE LEARNING

Interactive Patient
http://medicus.marshall.edu/medicus.htm

Virtual Autopsy
http://www.le.ac.uk/pathology/teach/VA

A product that takes full advantage of the multimedia nature of the Web is the Interactive Patient, developed by Marshall University School of Medicine. Visitors to this site can undertake a 'virtual consultation'. Beginning with a patient history—where you can ask questions via your computer keyboard to try and identify the illness—the program develops into one where you can examine various laboratory results and X-rays, and perform a virtual physical examination. Within the physical examination you have the option to inspect, palpate or auscultate the patient. If, for example, you auscultate the heart

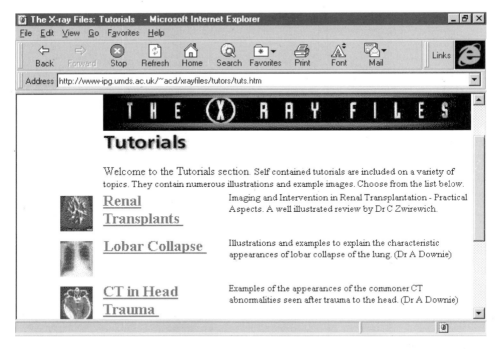

Figure 10.2   **Online tutorials at 'The X-ray Files'**

(by mouse-clicking on the appropriate part of the patient's torso) this sound will be downloaded and played on your computer. After reviewing the diagnostic evidence you are invited to submit a diagnosis and a course of treatment from a defined list. Visitors who correctly diagnose the condition receive a CME credit of one hour, awarded by the American Medical Association.

In contrast, staff at the University of Leicester have created the virtual autopsy Web site. Selecting from a list of seven self-contained cases, visitors are presented with a clinical history and a list of other signs and indicators. To help identify the cause of death, images of the patient's organs and post-mortem reports are presented for analysis. When all the evidence has been studied, visitors can select from a list the actual cause of death. If you get the answer wrong, there are additional hints to help you find the right one.

MEETINGS AND CONFERENCES

Doctor's Guide to the Internet — Meetings and Conferences
http://www.pslgroup.com/MEDCONF.HTM

Database of CME Events
http://omni.ac.uk/cme/search-cme.html

Perhaps the most popular way health professionals further their medical education is by attending meetings and conferences. To help physicians identify meetings of potential interest various services have started to appear on the Internet. The Meetings and Conferences section of the Doctor's Guide to the Internet provides a listing of over 5000 events in 84 countries. Events can be viewed by subject and by date/location, or if you seek a meeting on a specific topic then a search can be undertaken. Each entry in the database provides contact details (phone, fax and e-mail), event dates and the name of the sponsor or organizer.

For a more UK perspective, the Database of CME Events can be searched. Compiled by the Royal College of Physicians this database contains details of meetings that have been approved for CME. For example, a neurologist searching this database for forthcoming conferences on Parkinson's disease will find several relevant meetings, with details of fees and how many CME credits attendance will earn. Although currently only RCP-approved events are included, in the next few months it is hoped that other Royal Colleges will submit their approved events to this database.

REFERENCES

1   <URL: http://cancertrials.nci.nih/gov/> [Accessed 13 April 1998]

2   Hypertext links to Web sites of the various Royal Colleges are available at <URL: http://omni.ac.uk/cme/colleges.html> [Accessed 13 April 1998]

Quality of medical information on the Internet

After the recent US Food and Drug Administration approval of Viagra (sildenafil), the male erectile dysfunction drug, several Web sites came online and began marketing products with names such as 'Vaegra' and 'Viagro'. Though these were in reality nothing more than herbal supplements, by using a similar sounding name and citing the promotional data published by Pfizer Pharmaceuticals the purveyors were trying to mislead potential patients[1]. When Pfizer began filing law suits, these Web sites quickly disappeared.

More distressing are the Web sites that offer 'miracle cures' to people with chronic diseases. The Web pages of the Royal Rife Research Society, for example, have details of an electromagnetic 'frequency instrument' that can destroy cancer, and 'nearly every affliction known to man'[2]. Moreover, it is 'rapid, completely harmless [and has] no side effects'. In one study, or so the site informs the reader, 'every patient recovered without side effects of any kind'. Details of the study are vague, and a search of the MEDLINE database (1966–April 1998), CancerLit and the Cochrane Library yields no mention of the research Rife conducted or any clear evidence to support the claims made by this site.

These two examples demonstrate the potential danger of using the Internet as a source of medical information. However, this does not mean we should stop using the Internet. Just as we appraise stories we read in our newspapers — perhaps giving more credence to an editorial in *The Times* than we would to a reader's letter in a tabloid newspaper — we need to apply the same methodologies to the resources we find on the Internet. With this purpose in mind this article highlights several tools you can use to help ensure that you — or your patients — are not subjected to inaccurate or fraudulent medical information on the Internet.

QUALITY SEARCH FILTERS

OMNI
http://www.omni.ac.uk

Health on the Net
http://www.hon.ch/

Research undertaken by RelevantKnowledge shows that the most visited sites on the Internet are the big non-subject-specific search tools such as Yahoo! and Excite[3]. Though these search tools can be useful, their functionality for retrieving medical information is somewhat limited, for the reasons set out below:

- Too many resources are retrieved. Even when searching for the relatively rare condition 'juvenile arthritis' Excite still identified over 600 Internet resources

- No quality filters are applied. As search engines try to index as much of the Web as possible (large indexes attract a large number of visitors which in turn ensures that the owners can charge high rates for their advertising space), any search is likely to retrieve a mix of authoritative, speculative, and dubious information. Sifting the good from the bad can be difficult and time-consuming

Such problems can be negated by using specialty search tools, such as OMNI and Health on the Net, that have predetermined quality filters. For example, resources only get included in the OMNI database if 'they contain substantive information, of relevance to the OMNI user community. Personal pages or simply collections of pointers to other resources do not meet this requirement and are *de facto* excluded'. A detailed evaluation checklist provides further guidance on how sites are selected[4].

The Health on the Net Foundation have devised their own 'HONoured database' which includes *only* those resources that comply with the Foundation's Code of Conduct. Central to this code is the requirement that any medical information or advice hosted on a Web site must be authored by 'medically/health trained and qualified professionals'. If this condition can not be met then there must be a 'clear statement . . . that a piece of advice offered is from a non-medically/health qualified individual or organisation'.

Details of the search capabilities of these two services can be found in Chapter 1.

CRITICAL APPRAISAL

One of the underlying attractions of the Web is the way you can move seamlessly from one Web site to another, simply by following a hypertext link. However, in doing this it is easy to move from a quality-assured resource to a site where the data may be less reliable or even inaccurate. Consequently, as you navigate through the Web you must keep your critical faculties about you. According to Silberg[5] this appraisal can be distilled to four basic questions:

- Are the authors of the Web site clearly stated, along with details of their affiliations and credentials?

- Is the owner of the Web site prominently displayed, along with any sponsorship or advertising deals that could constitute a conflict of interest?

- Are any claims made by the site supported by research findings, and if so are details given to the original source of this data?

- Does the Web page contain details of when it was created and last updated?

If the answers to these questions are not readily available — or not disclosed at all — then any medical/health information given at such sites should be disregarded.

CURRENT INITIATIVES

Health Information Technology Institute
http://www.mitretek.org/hiti/showcase/index.html

MedPICS
http://www.derma.med.uni-erlangen.de/medpics/index.htm

Several initiatives, once developed, may greatly reduce the amount of inaccurate, dubious, and fraudulent health information on the Internet. The Health Information Technology Institute has devised a detailed set of criteria for measuring the quality of any medical Web site. Though this work is still ongoing, HITU hope to produce a checklist that will allow you to assign a score to any Web site. Sites that scored below a defined threshold would be deemed unsuitable as a source for health information.

A more revolutionary approach to quality is being developed by a team of German doctors who have devised medPICS. Based on the PICS (Platform for Internet Content and Selection) standard — originally devised to protect minors from accessing 'adult' sites — medPICS uses electronic tags as a way of filtering the medical information you retrieve from

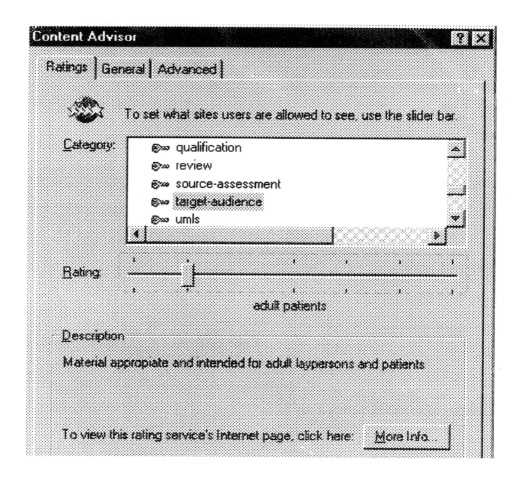

Figure 11.1 **medPICS—defining the target audience**

the Internet. These electronic tags could, for example, indicate who the intended audience is (consumers or professionals), whether the information is educational or promotional, and for which countries the information is suitable. Personal preferences are defined within your Web browser (Figure 11.1).

If this initiative succeeds — and organizations such as the American Medical Association and the World Health Organization agree to become independent rating bureaux — every time you subsequently access a medical Web site the medPICS filter would check to see what labels had been assigned. Dependent upon what these were, and how the browser has been configured, the filter could either block access to the site or display some disclaimer or warning.

REFERENCES

1   Ostom C. For new impotence drug, success breeds imitators. *Seattle Times* 22 April 1998. <URL: http://www.seattletimes.com/sbin/iarecord?NS-search-set=/354c4/aaaa003.d4c4698&NS-doc-offset=1&> [Accessed 2 May 1998]

2   <URL: http://www.rrrs.com> [Accessed 28 April 1998]

3   <URL: http://www.relevantknowledge.com/Press/release.html> [Accessed 28 April 1998]

4   <URL: http://www.omni.ac.uk/agec/evalguid.html> [Accessed 28 April 1998]

5   Silberg J. Assessing, controlling and assuring the quality of medical information on the Internet: *Caveat Lector* — let the reader and viewer beware. *JAMA* 1997;**277**:1244–5

The Internet and healthcare — the future

In his submission to the US Patent Office in 1876, Alexander Graham Bell wrote, 'there are many other uses to which these instruments [telephones] may be put, such as the simultaneous transmission of musical notes, differing in loudness as well as in pitch'[1]. With hindsight — and the development of new technologies — the idea of listening to a concert over the telephone is absurd. With this lesson in mind, speculation about how the Internet will be used in the next millennium should be treated with caution.

In the more immediate future, however, new health-related Internet applications are being developed and tested. This chapter will focus on these and consider the impact they may have on the delivery of effective healthcare.

DECISION-SUPPORT SYSTEMS

DXplain

http://www.lcs.mgh.harvard.edu/dxpdemo/start.htm (Demonstration)

Webweaver

http://www.med.virginia.edu/~wmd4n/medweaver.html

Since the advent of MEDITEL in the early 1970s, health professionals in the developed world have been using computerized decision support systems to facilitate the diagnostic process. Several of these products have appeared on the Web, and thus become available to any Internet-connected health professional, anywhere in the world. One system that can be accessed in this fashion is DXplain.

Developed by Massachusetts General Hospital, DXplain is a decision support system that uses a set of clinical findings — signs, symptoms and laboratory data — to generate a ranked list of diagnoses. When a diagnosis is offered, DXplain provides clinical reasons as to how this decision was reached, suggests what further clinical information should be collected to support the diagnosis, and lists any clinical manifestations that would be unusual or atypical for each of the specific diseases.

The system is accessed through a Web-based form where all clinical findings or manifestations that are deemed relevant are input. As terms are entered the DXplain system may suggest alternative, broader or narrower concepts to help focus the diagnostic query. (Though the term 'fever' is acceptable, DXplain has six narrower and more precise terms in its database.) When all the findings have been entered, the user clicks on the 'List Possible Diseases' button. For example, on inputting the findings, hip-pain, fever, growth retardation, chin recession, spleen enlargement and child, DXplain calculated that there was sufficient information to 'strongly support' a diagnosis of juvenile arthritis. The DXplain system justifies how this decision was reached—chin recession 'very strongly supports' this diagnosis—and provides additional information about the disease along with a list of bibliographic references for further reading. A paper by Johnson[2] that assessed the usefulness of the DXplain system in suggesting plausible diagnostic hypotheses reported that, 'in most cases, the DXplain program listed the correct diagnosis or a closely related diagnosis'.

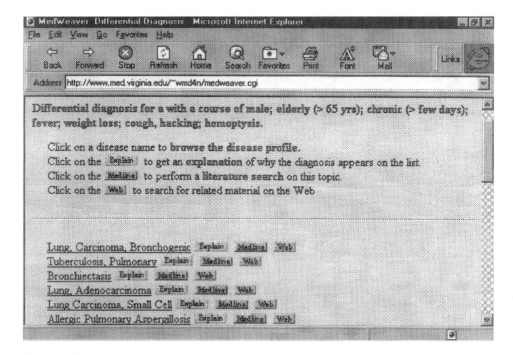

Figure 12.1   **Webweaver—integrating decision support, MEDLINE, and web searching**

Internet access to DXplain is currently in beta phase and is restricted to medical institutions or licensed physicians. Details of how to obtain a free user-name and password are available from the Web site listed above.

Another useful Web-based tool is WebWeaver. Developed By Bill Detmer of Stanford University School of Medicine, this product combines decision support (DXplain), MEDLINE literature searching, and exploration of the Web into a single application.

Though at present this product is only a prototype, the three cases available demonstrate its potential. For example, on selecting the case of the elderly male patient with 'several months of fever, weight loss, hacking cough, and coughing up blood' the decision support tool DXplain suggests various diagnoses including 'lung carcinoma bronchogenic'. At this point the WebWeaver software intervenes and offers the user an opportunity to seek an explanation of why this diagnosis was suggested, run a MEDLINE search on this topic, or search the Web for related material (Figure 12.1). By integrating these three features, WebWeaver acts as a 'one-stop' clinical information system.

INTERNET TELEMEDICINE

Armed Forces Institute of Pathology
http://www.afip.org/telepathology/index.html

Interactive Teaching Project in Surgery
http://av/ucl.ac.uk/tltp/

Next Generation Internet Initiative
http://www.ngi.gov/apps/

Internet telemedicine can take many forms. At a basic level the Internet can be used to forward — by e-mail or File Transfer Protocol — X-rays, pathology slides, or electrocardiograms from one doctor to another, to seek a second opinion or a more expert diagnosis. At a more advanced level, high speed Internet networks can be used to connect geographically remote health professionals in live, real-time teleconsultations.

The Armed Forces Institute of Pathology (AFIP), with 125 pathologists working in 22 subspecialties, is a world leader in the practice of pathology. Using e-mail or FTP this expertise can now be called upon by pathologists throughout the world. To make use of this service pathologists need access to a microscope with a high resolution camera, and image capture board and software to manage the images. These images are sent as e-mail attachments, or uploaded on the AFIP FTP site. On receipt of the image, AFIP aim to report the final diagnosis to the referring pathologist within 24 hours. No charges are made for consultations from US military establishments or for overseas contributors enrolled in military, WHO or other AFIP co-operative programmes. Civilian pathologists are charged $50 per consultation.

When sending an image by e-mail it is often necessary to use compression software to make the file smaller. Though this has an adverse effect on image quality, Della Mea[3] reported that pathologists who received the image by e-mail reached the same diagnosis in 85% of cases as those pathologists who saw the original images.

With the continuing development of high-speed networks in the UK—SuperJANET III for academics, NHSnet for NHS staff—remote interactive teleconsultations will become feasible. Already, medical students at six SuperJANET sites participating in the Interactive Teaching Project in Surgery can watch live operations and interact with the surgical team. In the United States networks that support broadband technology are being developed under the auspices of the Next Generation Internet Initiative. Medical Applications planned for this network include real-time telemedicine and remote-control telemedicine. The latter would allow the control of medical instruments from a distance, thus facilitating the development of robotic surgery.

Highly trained specialists are an expensive and scarce resource. Telemedical applications, such as those described here, help ensure that these resources are used effectively.

REFERENCES

1   United States Patent Office. Improvement in telegraphy. Alexander Graham Bell, of Salem, Massachusetts. Letters Patent No. 174,465, dated March 7, 1876 <URL: http://jefferson.village.virginia.edu. albell/bpat.2.html> [10 June 1998]

2   Johnson KB, Feldman MJ. Medical informatics and pediatrics. Decision-support systems. *Arch Pediatr Adolesc Med* 1995;**149**:1371–80

3   Dell-Mea V, *et al.* Telepathology using Internet multimedia electronic mail: remote consultation on gastrointestinal pathology. *J Telemed Telecare* 1996;**2**:28–34

Endpiece

A study, conducted in March 1998, calculated that the number of pages on the World Wide Web was around 275 million, and was growing at the rate of 20 million pages a month[1]. In an attempt to give a *flavour* of the eclectic nature of the Web, this final chapter describes a number of resources; some you may find useful and interesting, others may simply amuse.

The Voyeur in You?

http://voyeur.mckinley.com/cgi-bin/voyeur.cgi

If you have ever wondered what *other* Internet users search for, take a look at the Voyeur site. Updated every few seconds it provides a snapshot of the last few searches conducted on the Magellan Internet database. Any doubts about the popularity of the Spice Girls are very quickly dispelled!

Rail Planner

http://www.rail.co.uk

Developed by RailTrack this database of UK train times allows you to identify what trains are available, whether your journey will necessitate changing trains, and how long it will take to reach your destination. To search the database you simply enter your starting and destination stations, the date you wish to travel, and either the time you wish to depart or arrive by. For details of train services outside of the UK, the 'Trains and Railroads' section of the Yahoo! should be consulted. This can be reached by pointing your Web browser at http://www.yahoo.com/Business_and_Economy/Companies/Transportation/Trains_and_Railroads/

Internet Tutorials

http://www.netskills.ac.uk/TONIC/

If you have only recently started to use the Internet, and perhaps feel that you are not using it effectively, there are a number of Web-based tutorials at which you may want to look. The Online Netskills Interactive Course (TONIC) provides a good overview of the Internet with specific tutorials that focus on the types of networked information, the means for searching that information and an examination of the communication services available on the Net. Alternatively, visit the Yell Online Guide at: http://www.yell.co.uk/guides/explore/ index.html and read about more topical issues such as online banking and how to protect your computer from an Internet-borne virus.

Irreproducible Results
http://www.jir.com/

Describing itself as a source of 'timeless satirical and critique articles emanating from and about the scientific and medical community', visitors to *Journal of Irreproducible Results* Web site can read about the 'Triple-blind test' and how 'water can kill'.

Privacy on the Internet
http://www.13x.com/cgi-bin/cdt/snoop.pl

Though the topic of privacy on the Internet has received less media coverage than topics such as fraud or pornography, it is an issue that affects everyone who uses the Internet. Each time you visit a Web site you leave a 'footprint' that reveals where you have come from, what browser you are using, and what pages and files you have accessed. If you have enabled your browser to send and receive e-mail then your name and e-mail address can also be collected from your computer by prying Webmasters.

To draw attention to this issue the Center for Democracy and Technology (CDT) have created a privacy demonstration page where you can see what information your Web browser discloses about yourself. To run this demonstration point your browser at the address cited above.

Moments after visiting this site I received an e-mail message alerting me of the fact that I had visited the CDT site. At no point in the demonstration did I volunteer *any* personal information. As the CDT conclude, 'this is just one more example of how you can inadvertently provide information about you and your browsing habits as you surf the Net'.

Medical Clip Art
http://www.geocities.com/HotSprings/2497/

When presenting a paper or giving a lecture many health professionals use Microsoft PowerPoint or Harvard Graphics presentation software. Though both these products are good, the clip art graphics that are supplied with these applications are fairly predictable and very limited when it comes to medical images. One site on the Internet that addresses this problem is the Medical Clip Art site. This single site has over 100 medical clip art images including 'taking a tea-spoon of medicine', an 'asthma inhaler' and a 'happy doctor'.

Providing you are not going to use these images commercially, you can save any image and import it directly into your presentation.

Web Translation Service

http://babelfish.altavista.digital.com/cgi-bin/translate?

If you ever have the need to translate a document from one language to another there is now a free Web service you can use. The AltaVista translation service provides you with a tool to translate a grammatically correct document into something that is not necessarily perfect, but certainly comprehensible. Translations can be made from English to French, German, Italian, Portuguese and Spanish and vice versa. Figure 13.1 shows the results of a sentence written in German and translated into English.

E-MAIL TO FAX

Using a service devised by The Phone Company (TPC), it is now possible to send a fax via e-mail. To use this free service you simple need to address the e-mail message in the following way:

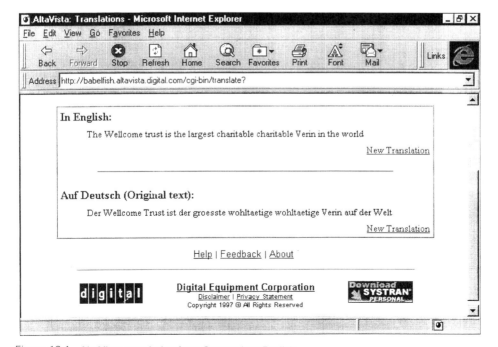

Figure 13.1   **AltaVista translation from German into English**

To: **remote-printer.***firstname_lastname@faxnumber***.iddd.tpc.int**

Replace the fields *firstname* and *lastname* with the name of the person you wish to fax and *faxnumber* with the appropriate number, prefixed with the appropriate (IDDD) country code. E-mail attachments (word processed files, etc) can *not* be sent via this service.

TPC is a volunteer organization that relies on 'local' Internet service providers to host a fax server and provide fax coverage for the local area. At present, coverage is available in 27 countries including the UK, USA and most of Australia. If you wish to check whether the destination you wish to fax to is covered by this scheme, point your browser at: http://www.tpc.int/verify.html

STATISTICAL ANALYSIS ON THE WEB

There are a number of Internet sites that can help clinicians with statistical analysis of their own research data. The Simple Interactive Statistical Analysis Web site (http://home. clara.net/sisa) enables visitors to perform *t*-tests, significance testing and so on by inputting data directly into a Web-based form (See Figure 13.2). Alternatively, if you wish to create customized data entry forms (perhaps based on a questionnaire) and undertake statistical analysis on these data, the Epi Info software can be downloaded from the Internet (http://www.cdc.gov/epo/epi/epiinfo.htm). Available without charge, this software comes complete with a manual and *free* technical support. Finally, if you require more information about statistics, statistical tests and study design, the 'Statistics at Square 1' text can be recommended. This item is available in full text at the *BMJ* Web site (http://www.bmj.com/statsbk/index.shtml).

URL Minder

http://minder.netmind.com/

The dynamic nature of the Internet means that keeping track of your favourite Web sites can be a time-consuming task. One utility, however, that can help minimize this workload is NetMind's URL Minder. Using a Web-based form you enter the URLs of the Web pages you wish to monitor. When the URL Minder detects that a page has changed — it may have been updated, moved to a different address, or have been deleted — you automatically receive a notification by e-mail. Depending upon the preferences that were defined when the URLs were initially registered, the mail message will contain either a link to the appropriate Web page or the updated page, delivered as a MIME attachment. No charges are levied to use this service.

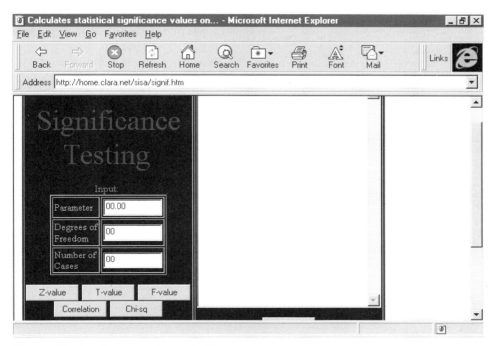

Figure 13.2 **Significance testing on the Web**

TRAVEL

If you are planning a foreign trip there are numerous sites on the Internet where you can check flight times and availability (http://www.british-airways.com/bookonline/), book hotels (http://www.hotelworld.com), and arrange car hire (http://www.avis.com/reserve-a-car/). One site that brings together a whole range of useful travel information is Yahoo! Travel (http://travel.yahoo.com). From these pages you can quickly identify the prevailing weather conditions, the current rate of exchange, and travellers' health information for numerous destinations throughout the world. A travel guide — from the *Lonely Planet* series — gives additional background information and a flavour of the country or city you intend to visit.

CONCLUSION

The resources available on the Internet are vast. This book has attempted to give you an insight into some of the more useful Web sites and Internet services, and in so doing demonstrate that, in the field of health and medical information, the Internet has lived up to the hype that surrounds this new electronic media.

Access to *all* the Web sites discussed in this book can be reached by pointing your Web browser at the Doctor's Internet Handbook home page: http://www.roysocmed.ac.uk/handbook.htm

REFERENCE

1   < URL: http://www.research.digital.com/SRC/whatsnew/sem.html > [Accessed 21 August 1998]

Index

access to site, blocking of 59–60
Accreditation Council for CME 52
addresses, list and listserver 27
Agency for Health Care Policy and
  Research (AHCPR) 34
AIDS and sexual health statistics
  49
AIDSDRUGS/AIDSLINE/
  AIDSTRIALS 23
alerting service, an 11
Allergy List Web archive 28, *28*
alphabetic browsing 4
AltaVista 1, *2, 6,* 69
AMA *see* American Medical
  Association
American Association for the
  Advancement of Science 22
American College of Rheumatology
  43
American Heart Association site 48
American Medical Association
  (AMA) 5
American Psychological Association
  21
Annals of Internal Medicine 37
Annual Review of Immunology 36
appraisal of information 31, 59
*Archives of Pediatrics and Adolescent
  Medicine* 5
Archives series of AMA 12
Armed Forces Institute of Pathology
  65–6
'arthritis', example of search for 26
Arthritis and Rheumatism Council
  for Research 22
Asian journals 16
asthma information 37, 50
authorship of site 59
autopsy online, virtual 53
Awards Almanac 22

Bandolier 33
banking online 68
Bell, Alexander Graham 63
BIOETHICSLINE 19, 21
biomedical resources 4, 13
Blood 38
Boolean operators 14
breast cancer articles 38
briefing papers 33
British Diabetic Association 3
British Journal of General Practice 43
British Medical Journal 3, 11, 12, 35,
  37, 70
browsing 1, 4, 60
  in electronic newspapers 8
  three methods of 4
BS 5750 (British Standards) 2

Canadian Clinical Practice
  Guidelines Infobase 33
'cancer', examples of search for 3,
  20, 33
Cancer Mondial Web site (IARC)
  48
Cancer Research Centre Web site
  3
cancer statistics 48, *49*
CANCERLIT 20, *20,* 57
car hire 71
cardiovascular diseases statistics 48
CD-ROM databases 13
CDPC *see* Communicable Disease
  and Prevention Control
CDSR *see* Cochrane Database of
  Systematic Reviews
CDT *see* Center for Democracy and
  Technology
Cell 36
Center for Democracy and
  Technology (CDT) 68
Centers for Disease Control 11
Cephalalgia 10
charges for services 8, 9, 10, 12, 22,
  42, 52, 66
  free 11, 13, 16, 19, 22, 25, 35,
    37
Charities Aid Foundation (UK)
  41–2
children, conditions affecting 42
choosing a service 6
citations, up-to-date additions of
  new 7, 11, 12, 14
'CJD', examples of search for 14,
  15, 49
classified topic browsing 5–6
Clinical Query Filter (in PubMed)
  14
CliniWeb 5–6, *6*
clip art, medical 68–9
'cloning', examples of search for 8,
  8
CME *see* education, continuing
  medical
Cochrane Collaborative Review
  Group headings 16
Cochrane Database of Systematic
  Reviews 14, 16, 33, 57
Code of conduct 2–3, 58
Cohen syndrome description *42*
Communicable Disease Prevention
  & Control 10, 50
communication, personal 25
compliance with Code of Conduct
  3
compression software 66
conferences 55–6
consultation, virtual 53–4

consumers (patients), health
  information for 41
Contact-a-Family (UK) 41–2, *42*
Coronary Prevention Group site
  48
cost *see* charges for services
credits in education *see* examinations
Creutzfeldt–Jakob disease (CJD)
  statistics 49
criteria of quality 4–5
current awareness 11–12
'cybersex' on Internet 21
'cystic fibrosis', example of search
  for 34

data entry forms, customized 70
database 3
  appointments 38
  dynamic links with related
    databases 14
  special collections and books 37,
    38
  supplemental data not in paper
    version 37
  three most popular 13
  traditional 7
  see also citations
Database of Abstracts of Reviews of
  Effectiveness (DARE) 22
Database of CME Events 55
Decision-support systems 63–4
Department of Health Web site 3
developments, keeping abreast of 7
'diabetes', examples of search for
  5
'diabetic retinopathy', resources on
  6
diagnosis online, virtual 53, 63–4
Directory of Mailing Lists Database
  26
discussion lists 25–6, *26*
Doctor's Guide to the Internet:
  Meetings and Conferences 55
Doctor's Guide Web site 10
Downie, Andrew 53
drugs information 23, 43–4, 57
DXplain 63–4

e-mail 9, 10–11, 25, 28, 36, 65–6,
  68
  to fax 69
EBM at McMaster University 31–3
education, continuing medical
  (CME) 51–5
Educational Grants Directory 22
effectiveness
  of discussion lists 28-9
  of health care and services 22

Effectiveness Matters Bulletin   33
electrocardiogram transfer   65
EMBASE   16
English language sources   13
Epi Info software   70
epidemics statistics   49, 50
'erectile dysfunction', example of
   search on 10, 57
ethics *see* code of conduct
European journals   16
evaluation of resources for inclusion
   in database   5
Evidence Reports (AHCPR)   34
evidence-based health discussion list
   28
evidence-based medicine   31–4, 37
examination and accreditation
   51–2
   membership and fellowship   52–3
examination of patients, virtual
   physical   53–4
Excerpta Medica database *see*
   EMBASE
Excite site   7, 58

FAQ (frequently asked questions)
   25–9
fax via e-mail   69
fees *see* charges
File Transfer Protocol   65
filtering medical information
   59–60
FIND-SVP report   41
flight times   71
FRCR examinations   52–3
funding   22
future of Internet and healthcare
   63

general health news   10–11
'genetic screening and health
   insurance', search for   19
Genome Database (Johns Hopkins
   University)   14
GLOBO*Can* statistics   *49*
GP-UK discussion list   25, 28
grants *see* funding
Grants Register   22
GrantsNet database   22
Guardian, The   8
Guide to Clinical Preventive Services
   34
gynaecology   32

Health Communications Network
   (Australia)   14
Health Information Technology
   Institute   59
Health of the Nation   43
Health on the Net (HON)   2, 6, 58
Health Services Technology
   Assessment Text database   34
Health Touch   42–3
HealthGate   21

Healthtel   4
heart attack survival calculator   32,
   33
heart disease and stroke
   statistics   48
HON *see* Health on the Net
hotel bookings   71
*How to Read a Paper: the Basis of
   Evidence Based Medicine (BMJ)*   37
Howard Hughes Medical
   Institute   22
Human Gene Mutation Database
   (Cardiff University)   14
hypertext links   35, 38, 59

Index Medicus   13
indexing,
   at individual page level   5-6
   large indexes   58
   of Medical Matrix Project   4
   MEDLINE database   31
   speed of   11, 14
information,
   for consumer   41
   critical appraisal of   59
   'fatigue syndrome'   7
   high quality   2, 5
   inaccurate or fraudulent   57
   irrelevant or misleading   1, 57
   overload   28, 58
   specific background   13
   too much   28, 58
initiatives, current   59–61
interactive learning   53–4
Interactive Patient   53–4
Interactive Teaching Project in
   Surgery   65
interests, special   26–7, *26*
International Agency for Research in
   Cancer   48
Internet search services   6

Jenkins, Dean   52
joining a list   25–6, 27
*Journal of the American Medical
   Association*   5, 11, 12, 37
Journal of Clinical Investigation   35,
   36, 38
Journal of Irreproducible Results   68
journals
   electronic   35–9
   epidemiological   50

keyword searches   8, 12

Lancet, The   11, 38
languages, foreign   69
leaflets for patients   43
legal judgments   19, 57
libraries, medical   13
Liszt (Microsoft mailing list)   *26,*
   26–27
Lonely Planet travel guide   71

McMaster University, Canada   31
Magellan Internet   67
Mailbase   27
mailing lists   26
mapping facility (translation of
   terms)   5
Marshall University School of
   Medicine   53
Massachusetts General Hospital   63
'measles', resources on   6
Medical Journal of Australia   36
Medical Matrix Project   4–5, *6*
Medical Sciences Bulletin   23
Medical Subject Headings (MeSH)
   5
Medicines Control Agency Web site
   3
MEDITEL   63
MEDLINE database   7, 11, 13–14,
   15, 16, 19, 21, 38, 57
MedPICS   59–60, *60*
Medpulse newsletter   10
Medscape   10
   CME   51–2
meetings and conferences   54–5
MeSH *see* Medical Subject Headings
messages, sending   25, 27
Micosoft Internet Explorer browser   1
'migraine', examples of search for
   1, 2, 10, 44
MIH Consensus Development
   Program   51
Miscarriage Association   42
misleading information   1
Morbidity and Mortality Weekly Report
   11, 50
MRCP Part 1 Question Bank   52,
   53

National Academy Press
   (Washington, USA)   35
National Asthma Campaign   50
National Back Pain Association   22
National Cancer Institute (NCI)
   20
National Center for Health Statistics
   (US)   47–8
National Institute of Allergy and
   Infectious Diseases   50
National Institutes of Health
   (NIH)   51
National Library of Medicine
   UMLS   14
   metathesaurus   5, 14
National Organisation for Rare
   Diseases (NORD)   42
National Organization for Rare
   Diseases (US)   41–2
Nature Medicine   12
NCI *see* National Cancr Institute
NetMind's URL Minder   70
Netscape Navigator browser   1
New England Journal of Medicine   7,
   12, 38

New NHS: A Modern Dependable, The (White Paper)   41
New Scientist   7
New York Times, The   8
news, general health   10–11
NewsPage (electronic newspaper) 7–9, *9*
NewsTracker (electronic newspaper) 7–9, *8*
newspapers, personalized electronic 7–9, *8*
Next Generation Internet Initiative 65, 66
NHS Centre for Reviews and Dissemination, York University 22, 33
NHSnet   66
NIH *Consensus Development Reports and Statements*   34
NLM *see* National Library of Medicine
Nuffield Foundation   22

obstetrics   32, *32*
Office of National Statistics (UK) 47–8
OMERACT   26
OMIM *see Online Mendelian Inheritance in Man*
OMNI *see* Organised Medical Networked information
oncology resources at Medical Matrix   3, *4*
'one-stop shop' resource   3, 12, 33
Online Mendelian Inheritance in Man 14, *15*
Online Netskills Interactive Course (TONIC)   67
online registration   4, 16, 21, 38
Oregon Health Sciences Library   5
Organised Medical Networked Information   4, 6, 58
'osteomyelitis', example of search for   11
'osteoporosis', example of search for   43
OVID Medline database (CD-ROM) 11
owner of site   59

page level index of resources   5
patients *see* consumers
PDF (portable document format)   38
Pediatrics   38
personalizing information   7–9
Pfizer Pharmaceuticals   57
Pharmaceutical Information Network (PharminfoNet)   23
pharmcology   16
Phone Company, The (TPC)   69
Platform for Internet Content and Selection (PICS)   59–60

POEMS (Patient Oriented Evidence that Matters)   33
population statistics   47
portable document format *see* PDF
practice guidelines, clinical   33
Pre-MEDLINE   14
press releases   10
Primary Care Clinical Effectiveness Team (Gwent)   33
privacy   68
problems of searching   1
Prostate Cancer Review   33
psychiatry   16
psychology   21
PsycINFO   21–2, *21*
publishing, traditional   7, 35
PubMed, MEDLINE   14, 35

Quality Health Inc Web site   1
quality search filters   6, 58
Question bank online   52

Rail Planner site   67
ranking system of Medical Matrix   4–5
registration, online   4, 16, 21, 38
RelevantKnowledge   58
research
    findings   11–12, 19, 33, 59
    funding   22
retrieval   7, 58
Reuters Health   10
reviews   14–16, 22, 33
Royal Rife Research Society   58

Science   38
Scottish Health Education Board site   43
searching   1, 5, 6, *6*
    appointments database   38
    comprehensive   6
    full text   38
    literature   11, 13
    quality filters   6, 58
    restricting categories   14
    sophisticated   14
    targeting strategy   8
    'Topic Search' (CANCERLIT)   20, *20*
self-help groups   41–4
Simple Interactive Statistical Analysis site   70
single source for many sites   11
slides, transfer of pathology   65
Society for Counselling and Information on Miscarriage   42
speed of electronic updating   11, 67
statistics   47–50, 70
    disease-specific   48–50
    vital   47–8
Statistics at Square 1 (BMJ)   37, 70
subject heading browsing   5

'sumatriptan', example of search for 23, 44, *44*
SuperJANET III   66
support groups *see* self-help groups
Surginet   26

tags, electronic   59–60
telemedicine, Internet   63–6
thesaurus (metathesaurus)   5
train services   67
translation
    from natural language to correct heading   5
    Web service for   69
travel   71
trials, clinical   31–2
TRIP *see* Turning Research into Practice
tuberculosis, search for   6
Turning Research into Practice (TRIP)   33, *34*
tutorials online   *54*, 67–8

UK Coronary Prevention Group   48
UK resources   3, 4
Ulrich's Periodicals Directory   31
UnCover Web   11–12
United Nations AIDS   49
URL Minder   70
US Food and Drug Administration 57
US Pharmacopeia   43, *44*
US resources   3

Viagra   57
VirSci Corporation   23
Virtual Autopsy site   53–4
viruses, computer   68
Voyeur site   67

Washington Post   8, 35
WebMedLit   11–12
Webweaver   63–4, *64*
Weekly Epidemiological Report   11
Weekly Epidemiological Report Web   50
Wellcome Trust   22
Whitaker's Books in Print   31
WHO Health Report 1997 (World) 47–8
WHO Statistical Information System (WHOSIS)   50
WISDOM — Sources of Biomedical Research Funding   22
Women's Health Initiative   43
World Health Organization   11
World Wide Web   67

X-ray Files   52–3, *53*, *54*
X-ray transfer   65
xenotransplantation issues   19

Yahoo! site   58, 67, 71
Yell Online Guide   68

NOTES

NOTES

NOTES